DETOX OUR BRAIN

10 Strategies for Brain Health and Wellness

SACHA LUCAS

MagletPublishing

ISBN: 978-1-7399248-2-9

Contents

Quiet the mind, and the soul will speak.

Ma Jaya Sati Bhagavati

Introduction

Our modern world is one of excess.

We have access to everything we could want, whether it's food, information, clothes or any other commodity. Because of this, we have an abundance of everything available to us. We buy too much food and waste even more. The fast-fashion industry allows us to buy a whole new wardrobe each year at a minimal price because we can just throw it out and do the same thing again next year when the threads start to unravel. Social media has indoctrinated us, leading us to believe that we need to keep our minds constantly engaged, flooded with information. We are convinced that we need to be available 24/7, that we need to see what all our friends are doing and posting online, otherwise we might miss out. We are flooding our minds and our bodies with an excess of everything, and we go to bed tired and heavy because of it. Our minds are still racing, filled with all the information we have put into it throughout the day, all the things we need to do tomorrow and in the coming weeks. How do we expect to wind down in a restful night of sleep when our minds are still processing all of that? The answer is, we can't. We then have a terrible night's sleep, and we wake up tired and lethargic and repeat the process the following day. It's unrelenting and exhausting.

This feeling of being heavy and stressed is probably something most of us relate to, but it's not a natural or healthy way to live. When our minds are cluttered, we suffer not only in our day-to-day living, but also in the long-term. You might find that you struggle to make decisions, and when you do, they often don't turn out to be the right ones. Because our minds never get a chance to rest and because they are filled to the brim with unnecessary information, anxieties, and stress, they don't function properly. Think of your mind like any other space in your home, like your kitchen or your office. If your kitchen is cluttered and filled with unnecessary things, how well does it function as a kitchen? If there are piles of clothes scattered across the counter and boxes all over the floor, will you be able to easily make meals and prepare food? Of course not! You'll take double the time to do anything because you have to keep moving things out of the way, creating space to actually chop and cook food. Your meal will take twice as long to prepare, and you might forget half of the ingredients because you can't find them. Your mind is the same. Like any other space, it functions best when it's uncluttered and organized.

I figured all this out when I was in my early 30s. I was working an office job at the time, with long and tiring hours, and I had no time in the day just for myself. I knew that I wanted to make something of myself, to keep progressing and moving forward—but I didn't know where I was going. I was single, didn't have any kids, and I wasn't spending the time I needed to figure out where I wanted to be. I was lost. I wasn't sure if I wanted to stay with the company and try to climb up the ladder through a series of promotions or whether I wanted to get out and do something different. But if I did want to do something else, what was it I wanted to do? I wasn't sure if I wanted a family or, if I did, when I did. I had all of these thoughts, feelings, and decisions racing around my mind, but I couldn't seem to get a grasp on any of them.

So I just kept going, working hard, and heading in a direction that I wasn't sure I even wanted to follow. I assumed that as long as I worked hard, whatever path I had found myself in would just work out for the best. I didn't really have a strategy or a plan beyond that. This wasn't just in my professional life, my evenings were flooded with activity too. I didn't spend my free hours on myself and my mental health, I spent them out socializing. I was out almost every night and drinking regularly. My diet was an afterthought, and sleep was not even on the list of priorities.

I don't know how long I would have kept going like this because at the time I didn't really recognize that I had a problem. This all changed when I went on vacation with a close friend of mine. We decided to take a full month off to go traveling throughout Europe, taking our time to explore everything from cities to small towns. It was a slow trip, one that was not rushed or filled with late nights and drinking. For the first time in a long time, I felt relaxed. I was getting enough sleep and rest, I was eating well, and I was keeping my body moving. I was also seeing new places and spending time connecting to new people with completely different life experiences than my own. It cleared my mind and my vision; I was truly able to see the world and myself. Brain fog that I didn't even know was there had been completely lifted. I started to take stock of my life and realized I had to change. I finally had the clarity to be able to make those decisions, and it led me to realize what I wanted to do.

When I got home, I decided immediately to quit my job, be proactive, and forge my own path. I started to live in a way that nourished my mind and my body, focusing on getting enough sleep, moving my body, and eating well. I rewired my mind, choosing to see the positive over the negative. I decluttered my life physically and learned to appreciate what I had. I found that through this, I was able to carry the focus and clarity I found on vacation into my everyday life, and I finally found a path for myself that had been so unclear just a few months earlier.

Decluttering your mind is an important action to take no matter your age or your situation. Everyone has a different experience, a different perspective, and a different way of dealing with things. You might have a higher tolerance for mental clutter than others or a lower one, but if your mental space is overwhelmed, then it's not functioning at its optimum level. A cluttered mind can manifest in several ways: it can lead to brain fog as well as heightened and uncontrollable levels of stress, anxiety, and depression. You might find that making decisions, for both everyday situations and life in general, has always been something you have struggled with. This is a major consequence of having a cluttered mind—you are unable to be confident in your decisions and you constantly feel like you are making the wrong one. Decluttering helps you to think clearly, to have a better memory, better cognitive functioning, and better problem-solving skills. You will feel that your mind is once again your own, and your body will feel back within your control too. The benefits of clearing your mind and body are countless, and you can experience them by following the strategies laid out in this book.

This is by no means a simple process, but it is a rewarding one. While it may seem like a giant, unapproachable task, the first step for any goal or life change is to break it down into smaller steps— and that's exactly what I have done for you. In this book, I have outlined the basics of what a cluttered mind is, how it can affect you, and the benefits of creating space and clearing it. This process has been made into 10 simple steps with strategies that you can easily start doing before you even put down the book. These are exercises that you can go through one by one to reach a state where you have worked through your clutter and your mind is clear. The pace at which you incorporate these strategies into your life is completely up to you! Some will be easier than others, it depends entirely on who you are as an individual.

The hardest part of any journey is the first step, but by choosing this book and making the conscious decision to declutter your mind, that's already out of the way! I will be with you for the rest of your journey, guiding you into a healthier and happier way of being. Everyone deserves to live a life unburdened and happy, and I'm going to help you to do that.

Your Cluttered Mind: What It Is, and the Damage That It's Doing

The most important parts of any journey are research and gathering information. If you don't fully understand what you're doing and where you're going, you're bound to get lost. Before setting out on a road trip, you make sure that you look at a map first to find the quickest route and all the possible pit stops along the way.

So, let's prepare for our journey. Before beginning the process of reducing your mental clutter, let's look at exactly what mental clutter is. In this chapter we're going to unpack exactly what it is we're looking to clear out. If we know what it is, how it manifests, and what causes it, it'll be far easier to tackle it.

What Is Mental Clutter?

Clutter is the same thing, whether it's in our room or our minds. It's a space that is disorganized and full of mess. It can come in any shape and form, and we can find it anywhere, from our kitchens to our poor, overused minds.

When a physical space in our home is cluttered, such as our bedroom or kitchen, we become less efficient doing anything in that room. It's harder to move around, to find things, or do anything because there is little space and lots of confusion. So, what do we do to remedy this? We spend time cleaning it out—we throw dirty clothes into the laundry, toss away old wrappers we find lying around, clean the dishes, dry them, and put them away again. We are constantly decluttering our physical spaces so that we can keep functioning in them optimally.

But we are not trained to do the same for our minds.

Mental clutter is simply that; the mess and disorganization that accumulates in our minds because we don't spend any time clearing it. When we have so much happening in our minds, our heads go into overdrive. We can't focus on thinking clearly because our minds are racing, trying to sort through everything that is taking up our mental space.

Mental clutter is a different experience for everyone, as our minds are all very different. However, there are several common ways that it can present, and you might relate to one or all of them. The first is an overload of information, which happens when having too much information to process has led to you feeling mentally drained. Second, it might be an overload of negative feelings, stress, anxiety, and depression that you carry around every day and cannot seem to shake. It can also manifest as procrastination. This is when you are putting off doing things that sit at the back of your mind, whether it's scheduling a doctor's appointment, doing laundry, or paying a certain bill. Because we put them off, the tasks stay rooted in our minds until we do them. Another way it can present itself is as high and specific expectations of the people in your life and the world around you. Do you find yourself frustrated when you want things a certain way and people don't follow along? Maybe it's how you think the towels should be folded, or the opinions of your friends and your family that you just don't agree with. Instead of understanding that everyone is different, it makes you angry and exasperated.

When we go through our days dealing with mental clutter, we tend to find ourselves constantly irritated, distracted, and down.

Three Main Types of Mental Clutter

Now that we know the basics of mental clutter, let's look at the three main ways that you may feel the effects of it in your everyday life.

Worry

Worry is ultimately the inability to focus on the present. Our minds wander to our future, and we think of all the worst possible scenarios. This is what it means to worry, and it's true whether we're worrying about the next day or 10 years into the future. On some level, we are attempting to prepare ourselves for some unknown event or negative event. Or perhaps we believe that by worrying we can prevent the undesirable outcome from happening. But instead of preventing the negative experience, what inevitably happens is that worrying just means going through something bad twice.

While it's not advisable to ignore the future, we don't need to attach negative feelings of anxiety and stress to trying to create the best outcome. These emotions stop us from seeing clearly, as our perception is tinted by worry. Mental clutter in the form of worry can often paralyze us, as all we can see is everything that could go wrong.

Guilt or Indecision Over Your Past

Our life is made up of a thousand choices, and one of the prominent ways that people experience mental clutter is indecision or guilt over the decisions that have already been made. When we constantly ruminate over the past, we stay in the past, and worrying about it stops us from enjoying the present. Similarly, feelings of guilt keep us rooted in the worry over decisions that are now history. Furthermore, we may think that we should have something different than we have, but we will never truly know where a different choice would have led. We always tend to think that there is a better life than what we have, but we can never know for sure. Allowing your mind to go around in circles of past decisions just leads to unnecessary despair. Mental clutter can force us to stay in the past because our minds are too chaotic to live in the present.

Negative Self-Talk

The last manifestation of mental clutter is consistent negativity. This is aimed especially at yourself and presents as negative self-talk or poor confidence. However, it can also be directed to your life and the people around you. If you find yourself often talking negatively to yourself, thinking that you are just the worst, or that you don't have worth—this is also a symptom of mental clutter. These thoughts and emotions of worthlessness tend to take space in our minds and add to the clutter. We often don't realize that we're doing it, and therefore, we don't change anything. But our thoughts influence our behavior and our actions, and we will not do what is best for ourselves because we don't believe that we deserve it.

Causes of Mental Clutter

There are many reasons why we build up mental clutter over time. To break down these habits you have to understand where they come from. There's no point in treating the symptoms of a disease without curing the causes, because until you fix the causes the symptoms will just keep popping back up.

Stresses of Daily Life

First and foremost of the causes of mental clutter, is stress. Persistent stress is the ultimate enemy of a healthy and happy life because it breaks down both our bodies and our minds. We can be stressed because of a number of things; it can be caused by work, school, our friends, our family, or even our own expectations of ourselves. It's when we feel overwhelmed and panicked, like we can't do everything, or we have too many things racing through our minds. While it's natural to be stressed at times, it should never be consistent or something that you are dealing with daily. Your body and mind are not equipped to deal with this level of stress for extended periods.

However, with the fast pace of our world these days, and the expectations that we place on ourselves, daily stress is common for most people. Stress causes us to overthink things, filling our minds with worries and anxieties which eventually causes mental clutter. Furthermore, it also can cause various health problems, such as headaches, insomnia, and a weakened immune system. These problems only serve to further aggravate mental clutter. Because our minds are overwhelmed with stress, we reach for negative coping mechanisms rather than addressing the source—stress and mental clutter. The only way we can reduce stress is by changing our lifestyle. The way we live is a significant factor in the extent of our mental clutter, and we will explore this in greater detail in Chapter 3.

Overwhelming Amount of Choice

The next root of mental clutter that we will be looking at is the paradox of choice that we have in modern society. Objectively, we have more freedom than ever. We go through life with thousands of choices: what we want to do for work, what to do with our free time, and even down to things we have to do every day, like choosing what to eat and what to wear. While having so much autonomy over our lives may seem positive, it has been shown that having too many choices, and having to make decisions constantly, can often lead to feelings of anxiety and being overwhelmed.

This is known as decision fatigue. It's the idea that after having to make too many choices all the time, we start to feel paralyzed because we have become tired, stressed, and unable to make decisions. These paralyzing decisions are not necessarily big choices—they include the small decisions you have to make every day, such as what to have for breakfast or which pair of jeans to buy. We live in a world of excess with more and more choices each day, and this only adds to feeling overwhelmed. Something as simple as going shopping for groceries requires more than a dozen decisions, as we have so many choices and so many things available. This leads to our minds becoming cluttered with all the choices we have made, regrets over some of those choices, and anxiety over all the choices we will have to make in the future.

The Negativity Bias

Our inherent tendency to react more strongly to negative stimuli than to positive ones is called the negativity bias. Our brains are quick to latch on to the negative things in our lives, the negative comments about us, and the bad things that are happening. Our brains are like Velcro with negativity; we process it faster, it has a bigger impact, and it tends to stick around for longer. This means that we frequently see all the negatives in a situation and within ourselves first. We see all the ways we fall short and all the ways we could fail long before we recognize our talents and imagine the best scenario.

This leads to increased stress and exacerbates mental clutter. To declutter our minds, we have to rewire this part of ourselves.

Physical Clutter and Excess

Lastly, one of the greatest contributors to mental clutter is physical clutter. At the end of the day, our mind is a reflection of our environment. Just as we start to reflect the people around us in our thoughts and behaviors, if your space is overwhelmed with things, your mind will start to mimic this too.

This is true for your physical space, like your room, apartment, or house, and it's even true for your online spaces. When your phone is full of messages, notifications, and social media applications that you feel obligated to check every day, that too is a form of clutter.

In our physical space, we also tend to hold on to an excess of things. Capitalism has trained us to buy more of everything than we could ever need, whether it's clothes, food, jewelry, devices, and anything else. But the more stuff that we have, the more daily decisions that we have to make. Physical clutter makes it harder for us to operate smoothly in our spaces because we cannot move around freely. Furthermore, our constant need to be available online and to not miss out on anything overloads our minds. All this excess leads to mental clutter.

Effects of Mental Clutter

The effects of mental clutter are destructive to our short- and long-term happiness and health. It makes our minds foggy and prevents us from thinking clearly as well as impacting on our productivity and making it hard to focus or get anything done. It can lead to irritability and mood swings, as we become so overwhelmed by everything that any small thing is hard to handle. But your mental health is not the only thing that suffers. While the detrimental effects of stress will be felt in your mentally and emotionally, physically it's actually harming the tissues of your brain. The chronic stress that is caused by mental clutter can make you vulnerable to mental health problems, cause memory loss, and even has the potential to change your brain structure if left untreated for too long. Chronic stress also kills your brain cells and shrinks your brain matter, which inhibits memory, learning, and emotional control centers. Stress physically breaks down your brain, and if it is left for years, the effects of this will follow you for the rest of your life.

Mental clutter is detrimental not only for our mind but for our bodies too because of the chronic stress that it induces. Stress affects all of the major systems that maintain balance throughout our body, such as the central nervous system, endocrine system, respiratory, and vascular systems. It causes havoc in your body by unbalancing these systems, as the extra cortisol that is being released when you are stressed triggers different responses throughout your body. It damages your respiratory system because it causes your heart to beat faster, constricts your blood vessels, and it can trigger high blood pressure.

Your endocrine system is in charge of hormone regulation throughout your body; however, chronic stress will secrete more of some hormones while inhibiting others. When the balance of our hormones is disrupted, it throws everything into disorder, including your digestive system. This is why stress can often cause us to have stomach problems. Stress also causes your muscles to tense up, preparing for action, but if your stress is chronic, they never get a chance to relax. This can cause muscle aches and pains as well as headaches and can stop you from exercising or getting through the day pain-free. Furthermore, an imbalance in your hormones can play havoc with your appetite as well as cause high blood pressure, and can lead to issues with drug and alcohol abuse as it affects your ability to make decisions.

Our bodies and minds function best when balanced, and mental clutter completely disrupts any balance that we could potentially have. If left for years or decades, you can get to a point where it is impossible to reverse the damage. To look out for your future health, as well as feel better in your everyday life, it's essential to clear the clutter from your mind. Life is too short to be suffering through your days.

2

A Closer Look Inside Your Mind: Introduction to the Glymphatic System

One of the first things that you need to understand before attempting to declutter your mind, is the glymphatic system. This is the system that our brain uses for clearing its waste. However, like any other part of your body, the optimal functioning of our glymphatic system is dependent on balance, on us leading a healthy lifestyle, and taking care of our bodies. Our glymphatic system also has a symbiotic relationship with our sleeping patterns, as they are dependent on one another. When we neglect sleep, our glymphatic system suffers, and when our glymphatic system suffers, so does our sleep.

We will spend this chapter exploring the glymphatic system in more detail—looking at what it is and how it functions. Most importantly, we will break down exactly how neglecting it can contribute to mental clutter. Neglect of the glymphatic system and mental clutter are intrinsically linked, and in order to understand the roots and cures for mental clutter better, you need to understand your glymphatic system first.

The core function of your glymphatic system is to remove toxins and waste from your brain, thereby enabling it to keep running smoothly. As our cells undergo their normal function, they produce metabolic waste, a byproduct leftover from our cellular processes that cannot be used so it just lingers. For example, when our bodies convert food into energy, or other similar processes, byproducts such as carbon dioxide and sulfites are produced. Our body cannot use any of this, so they are just left in the gaps between the cells—also known as the interstitial space—and when the waste products are not cleared up it prevents our cells from functioning properly.

For the rest of the body, it is the job of the lymphatic system to clean up this waste. The lymphatic system is composed of several vessels and nodes throughout the body that help to clear out metabolic waste from between your cells. However, our central nervous system (CNS), which the brain is a key part of, does not have any lymphatic nodes or vessels. But the CNS is exceedingly active; it interprets all sensory information and essentially sends this information around to different parts of the body. Therefore, metabolic waste piles up in our CNS fairly quickly. The CNS is also an incredibly intricate and complex system, and small fluctuations in its environment can easily impede its natural function; therefore, any waste that builds up needs to be cleared away quickly.

So, if the lymphatic system has lymph nodes and vessels to clear up waste, what does the glymphatic system use? The answer is glial cells. These cells are as numerous in the CNS as neurons are, and they were previously thought to just be support for cells. Glial cells not only nourish and insulate neurons, they also play a key role in the glymphatic system removing waste from between the neurons. The most important glial cells for us are those known as astroglia, as they help the exchange of fluid, mainly cerebrospinal fluid, between the CNS and the glymphatic system. Cerebrospinal fluid is a clear liquid that surrounds the CNS, most importantly the brain. The glial cells channel this fluid into the CNS, allowing it to flow through the interstitial spaces, collecting toxins, proteins, and all other waste products that are collected around the cells. The fluid carrying the waste then flows back through the glial cells to the glymphatic system.

This exchange is supported by the fact that the glymphatic system runs parallel to our arteries. The rhythmic pulsing of the blood, and subsequent expansion of the blood vessels, help to keep things moving quickly. The glymphatic system then links up with the lymphatic system at the second membrane surrounding the CNS, and the metabolic waste is excreted from the body through the lymphatic system. A glymphatic system that does not function properly can lead to brain fogginess, memory loss, insomnia, and has been linked to several cognitive problems, including Alzheimer's disease (Reeves, Karimy, et al, 2020).

The glymphatic system functions mainly while we sleep, so it's also directly related to sleep quality. This is because when we sleep, the interstitial space in our CNS increases by approximately 60% (Newman, 2019) due to the effects of norepinephrine, which is a neurotransmitter produced in the brain. It's only produced when we're awake, and when it is produced, it causes swelling in the cells of the glymphatic system and inhibits the flow of cerebrospinal fluid. This means that the interstitial space is decreased and less fluid is flowing. However, when we sleep norepinephrine is not produced, our cerebrospinal fluid flows freely, and the space between our cells increases (Drew, 2020). This increased space allows for the cerebrospinal fluid to flow uninhibited through our CNS, which boosts the exchange of fluids and, therefore, the removal of metabolic waste. It's important not only that we get the right amount of sleep, but also that the sleep we get is of good quality.

The glymphatic system is the brain's very own detoxification system, essentially the personal garbage removal service for your mind. Your mind might be buzzing a bit at this point, and you may be wondering, how does this all link back to mental clutter? Well, when our glymphatic system is not functioning efficiently, our cognitive functioning suffers too. It can lead to brain fogginess, indecisiveness, bad memory, and slow processing—all of which are symptoms of mental clutter.

On a biological level, a poor functioning glymphatic system leads to an excess of metabolic waste in our minds. To declutter our mind on a mental level, we also have to declutter on a physical level; and understanding and fixing our glymphatic system is the only way to do this. Increased mental clutter can also interfere with the glymphatic system as it often leads to high blood pressure. High blood pressure can interfere with the removal of metabolic waste as it causes our blood vessels to lose their elasticity and become increasingly stiff. As previously mentioned, the arteries play a significant role in keeping the glymphatic system moving, as the expansion and movement of the blood vessels assist the exchange of fluids. This is slowed down if the blood vessels are stiff.

Sleep is linked to mental clutter as well as the glymphatic system. If our minds are cluttered, we do not sleep well, our blood pressure rises, stress slows our system, and our glymphatic system suffers. But the reverse is true, too—if our glymphatic system is not working well, we tend to have cognitive issues, and it can be harder to declutter our minds. The glymphatic system is intrinsically linked to mental clutter, and it's an essential function to understand as we make the move towards decluttering our minds.

Some of the best ways to support and maintain our glymphatic system is with a healthy lifestyle, a good diet, and regular exercise. However, the most important building block for a healthy system is sleep. In the next chapter, we will look at different ways to ensure not only that you get enough sleep, but also that your sleep is of good quality.

Three Basic Building Blocks of Health and Happiness

The foundation of good mental and physical health will always be a consistently healthy lifestyle, and this is also how you will start your recovery journey. Every few years there will be a brand-new health fix that 'guarantees' to solve all your problems with a two-week diet or a pill that balances all the issues in your gut. But none of these will ever work. To assist your glymphatic system and clear your mental clutter, a balanced lifestyle is key; and the three most important steps for a balanced lifestyle are: reliably good-quality sleep, a balanced diet full of whole foods, and keeping your body moving by exercising regularly and building physical activity into your normal daily life. It's also important to understand that these are all linked to one another. Like three legs that are holding up a table, if you don't focus on making sure all three are stable, the table will topple, as will your health.

As we move through the chapters of this book, you will be exposed to 10 different strategies that are designed to declutter your mind and improve your overall mental and physical health. However, these strategies will not be effective if you don't work on your lifestyle first. Think of this chapter as the foundation for the rest of the book and for the lifestyle you are aiming to build.

If you are exercising, you can sleep better; and if you are sleeping well and eating a balanced diet, then you will have the necessary energy to work out and keep your body moving.

The Importance of Good Sleep

In the previous chapter we briefly touched on the importance of sleep, particularly in relation to the glymphatic system. Without sleep, our minds can't be properly cleared of metabolic waste. Sleep is one of the easiest ways to detoxify not only our bodies, but also our minds. This detoxification process is essential for cleaning mental clutter, and neglecting this process can cause the cognitive functioning of our minds to dramatically decrease. Our minds get foggy, our memory is clouded, and it's impossible to function at an optimal level day-to-day if our minds are full of waste and rubbish.

But sleep is not important only for clearing the waste from our minds, it's also essential for the functioning of every system throughout our body because it affects the release of our hormones. For example, insomnia can often lead to weight gain. This is because lack of sleep affects the ghrelin and leptin hormones—the ghrelin hormone is responsible for creating your appetite, while the secretion of the leptin hormone signals you to stop eating (Mann, 2009). When we are sleep-deprived, our bodies secrete more of the ghrelin hormone and less of leptin, causing us to eat more without stopping, whether or not we are hungry. If this happens enough over time, it can cause steady weight gain. This is just one of the ways that lack of sleep disrupts the regular functioning of our bodies, but it tends to have a far bigger impact on our brains than any other organ.

Why Does the Brain Need Sleep?

Our brain uses the time we sleep for performing maintenance, repairing functions throughout the system, and making sure that everything is in good working order. It's a time for rest, not only for your body, but also for your mind, and as we know, rest is the essential period when we gather ourselves and ready ourselves for the next day. Why wouldn't our brains need time to do the same?

For example, one of the most important things our brains do while we sleep is consolidate and store our long-term memory, ensuring that our memories are kept safe. During the day, we create a mountain of knowledge and images, but not all of them are worth saving. Therefore, when we sleep, our brains sort through all the short-term memories we have made during the day and set aside the important ones to be transferred into long-term memory. It does this by strengthening the neural connections between the memories that need to be stored and pruning those that are unnecessary (Walton, 2016). This is the reason sleep is so essential when you're studying; it helps to secure the information you have learned into your head. It's also important for our memory capacity and recall skills in the long-term. If we are sleep-deprived, we'll not only struggle with memory on the days after we slept badly, but our brains will also start to lose the ability to store knowledge at all, further damaging our memory.

Sleep is necessary for boosting the cognitive abilities of our minds. This is probably something you have already noticed when you try and trudge through the day on a few hours of poor or interrupted sleep. Your brain gets foggy and processing doesn't happen nearly as fast or as easily as usual. There are dozens of studies that show how sleep deprivation kills our cognitive abilities, affecting everything from our logic to our decision-making skills. It especially impacts the higher cortical functioning of the brain, which is the part responsible for higher-level functioning such as awareness, vision, visual-spatial recognition, and multitasking (Killgore, 2010). Lack of sleep can also impact your ability to concentrate and your working memory. It has been shown that even a small but consistent deficiency in sleep can severely impact your attention span. A study has found that losing as little as two hours of sleep every night over 14 days significantly impacted the participants' ability to perform tasks that involved concentration and reasoning (Walton, 2016). Regular cognition and reasoning are not possible without a suitable amount of sleep; and if our minds cannot function properly, the clutter will continue to build up.

Sleeping also helps to boost our creativity, and lack of sleep interrupts certain types of thinking that are essential for the creative process. Most notably, it tends to break down neurodivergent thinking, which is essentially being able to think outside of the box. This includes finding new and imaginative ways of doing things, the ability to think flexibly, moving around a problem, generating original ideas, and fluency in thought patterns. Without sufficient sleep, our brains are unable to see things from a different perspective, and they get stuck in the same patterns.

Lastly, sleep deprivation can lead to several mental health problems, including depression and anxiety. There is an established link between lack of sleep and depression, in particular, both in causation and symptom. Those suffering from depression often have trouble with their sleep, whether they are sleeping too long or often or suffering from insomnia. However, it's also true that sleep deprivation can intensify feelings of depression, so it becomes a cycle where one just serves to worsen the other. One explanation for this is that depression tends to disrupt your circadian rhythm, which is the body's natural cycle in which all internal processes take place, including the regulating of sleep. Depression can be both a cause and a symptom for worsening mental clutter; therefore, learning to balance your sleep to maintain your mental health is an important step.

How to Improve Your Sleep

Sleep is clearly essential for the healthy functioning of our brains. So, what can we do to make sure that we get the right amount? There are many ways that you can improve your sleep, but as previously mentioned, it's not just the quantity of sleep that you need to focus on, but also the quality. The recommended amount of sleep an adult should aim to get each night is anywhere between seven and nine hours. Where you land in that range is a personal matter of how much sleep makes you feel your best. It's also important that your sleep schedule is consistent, i.e. that you go to bed at the same time every night and that you wake up the same time each morning. Irregular sleeping patterns not only disrupt our circadian rhythm, but also decrease our levels of melatonin, which is the hormone that signals the brain to begin sleeping (Mawer, 2020). If you are struggling to get to sleep, try being more consistent with when you sleep! Avoiding irregular or long naps is also an important part of maintaining your circadian rhythm. Short power naps can be beneficial, but sleeping during the day tends to disrupt your internal clock, making it harder for you to fall asleep at night. It can also leave you feeling groggy throughout the rest of the day. However, if you incorporate naps of 30 minutes or less into your everyday schedule, your body tends to get used to it. If you're having problems sleeping, though, it might be better to avoid naps altogether for the sake of your nightly slumber.

There are several lifestyle habits that you can adopt to improve the quality of your sleep. If you have severe sleep problems, it is a good idea to cut caffeine out of your diet, or at least ensure that you don't consume anything with caffeine past a certain time of day. While caffeine can have some benefits when it is consumed in the afternoon and later, it stimulates your CNS and can stop your body from relaxing at night and falling asleep easily. Caffeine can stay in your body for up to eight hours after you've had it, so it's advisable to stop drinking coffee and caffeinated teas after about 3 or 4 pm. In fact, some experts recommend avoiding caffeine after as early as 2 pm.

Alcohol can also disrupt your sleeping pattern, and cutting it from your diet can help, mainly because it disrupts the production of melatonin, making it hard to fall asleep or causing restless sleep. While you can have a glass of wine in the afternoon and you will most likely be fine, it's recommended to avoid drinking all types of alcohol later at night.

Another tip to improve your sleep is to expose yourself to natural light earlier in the day and prevent yourself from being exposed to blue light later in the evening. Natural and bright light throughout the day helps to regulate your circadian rhythm and increase your energy. It signals to your body that you are meant to be awake and active. You can either focus on getting daily sunlight exposure or invest in artificial sunlight bulbs. Similarly, darkness signals to our body that we need to sleep, as it stimulates the production of melatonin and helps to regulate your circadian rhythm. This natural sleep signal is completely disrupted when your brain is exposed to bright light late at night, especially the blue light emitted by our electronic devices. You can either find glasses that block blue light or make it your nightly routine to stop looking at all screens at least two hours before you go to bed. In fact, you should even move your phone to another room at night altogether. It has been found that having your smart phone in the same room where you sleep exposes you to high levels of radiation that emanate from your phone and that can cause dysfunction to your hormones and the biological rhythm that helps you sleep.

There are several little habits you can adopt in your night-time routine to allow your mind to wind down and prepare itself for sleep. Make sure not to eat late, as consuming food can disrupt your melatonin production. Create a routine and environment that makes you feel calm. Allow yourself one to two hours before bed to calm your mind, staying away from electronic devices.

Studies suggest that taking a warm bath or a shower just before bed helps you to relax your body and fall asleep faster, improving the quality of your sleep (Liao et al., 2005). Taking a hot bath before bed has been proven to boost sleep, as it causes your core body temperature to drop, and this drop signals to the brain that it is time to rest.

Other nighttime rituals that might help you wind down before bed are playing relaxing music, practicing breathing exercises, meditation, or reading a few chapters of your favorite book. Daily exercise and eating enough food are also important things you can do during the day that help to boost your sleep at night.

You can also create a bedroom environment that promotes sleep and doesn't interrupt it. You can do this by making sure there are no bright lights, that your room stays quiet throughout the night, and that the temperature is comfortable so that you don't wake up too cold or too hot. Make sure that your bedding is cozy and that your pillows fit your needs. The wrong pillow can create many problems with your back and neck, so make sure it's not too high or too low. Little adjustments like this can mean the difference between a satisfying, long rest and one where you wake up wondering if you ever actually slept at all.

Through these tips and tricks, you will be able to regulate and improve your sleeping pattern so that your body and mind have time to recuperate. This is only one of the steps that allow for the process of mental decluttering to be possible, but by following it you will see a significant improvement in your everyday life. Let's move onto the next one—diet.

The Role of Diet in Health

When we speak about the necessity of diet for your health, both mental and physical, the main focus is on getting in the macronutrients and micronutrients that your body and mind need to function at their best. After all, your body is basically a machine; you need to feed it fuel that will make it run smoothly. For example, if you want your car to run, you fill it up with fuel, don't you? If you decided instead to pour maple syrup into your gas tank, it wouldn't get very far, would it? Just like a car, our bodies need to be filled with the proper fuel to get moving. We need a balance of the three macronutrients every day (carbohydrates, proteins, and fats) as well as a wide variety of micronutrients in the form of vitamins and minerals, to function and feel our best. This is not only important for our bodies, but also immensely important for our minds. Our minds are fueled by what we eat, and if we don't offer it a variety of quality fuel, it's going to fall short.

Food has a far greater effect on our physical brain than we often realize. The building blocks of the food we consume determine how well our brain can function on a day-to-day basis. Certain diets nourish the brain; for example, a diet rich in vitamins, minerals, and antioxidants can boost your cognitive abilities as well as protect your brain from oxidative stress, which can damage brain cells. Diets rich in specific foods, such as the whole foods, healthy fats, nuts, and grains typically found in the Mediterranean diet, have even been proven to slow down the damaging effects of aging on the brain. It has been shown that this type of diet lowers the risk of cognitive impairment and decline while helping to prevent the development of dementia (van de Rest et al., 2015). Let's look at the specific impact each of the food groups has on the health of our brain.

Essential Food Groups for Balanced Brain Health

While carbohydrates have been attacked in the dieting industry in the last decade, they are actually essential for fueling our brain. While our brain makes up only 2% of our body weight, it consumes about 20% of the energy that carbs, specifically glucose, deliver to our bodies (Mergenthaler et al., 2013). Without this energy, our brains cannot function properly. This doesn't mean you should justify pancakes every morning to help you work better, but carbs are important! When carbohydrates are broken down, the glucose released plays an essential role in producing serotonin, which balances your mood and feelings of anxiety. Without carbohydrates, your brain will lack the energy to function, and you will find yourself emotionally unstable, and suffering from feelings of depression. It's important, though, to eat whole grain, complex carbohydrates like brown rice and starchy vegetables because simple carbs like white bread and sugar break down into glucose too fast, and your brain misses out.

Fat is the second macronutrient that your brain needs; but as there's a right kind of carbohydrate, it's also important to consume the right kinds of fat. You need to focus on having omega-3 fats, which are found mainly in fatty fish such as salmon and in olive oil. These fats are vitally important for the development of the brain in the womb and early childhood, and thereafter are necessary for the maintenance of a healthy brain. This is because they are essential for our cell membranes as well as the healthy functioning of neurons. In fact, around 60% of the brain is made of omega-3 fats! Because the body can't produce omega-3 fats itself, you have to provide them from food. Therefore, neglecting to include healthy fats in your diet can seriously affect your cognitive abilities and could lead to cognitive diseases, such as dementia, later in life.

Next, there is the role of probiotics, vitamins, and minerals. To understand the importance of probiotics, you first need to understand that there is two-way communication between your digestive tract and your CNS, and this is known as the 'gut-brain' axis. Basically, when your gut is healthy and processing properly, your cognitive function is regulated too. Probiotics help to keep your gut moving and regular and can be found in fermented foods, yogurt, or even in the form of supplements. Probiotics are specifically helpful in controlling mood disorders.

The various vitamins and minerals all have different roles that aid your brain's functioning. For example, vitamin E assists the transportation of messages to the cells, calcium is an important nerve cell transmitter, and vitamin C and certain B vitamins help form the nerves. Therefore, having a diet that is rich in a diverse range of vitamins and minerals is essential to keeping your operation running smoothly. You can ensure your body gets the necessary variety by eating a wide range of fruits, vegetables, and whole grains.

Last, but not at all least, is the importance of hydration. While drinking water is often praised for the health benefits it has for your body, it's equally beneficial for your brain. Even mild dehydration can significantly impact how well your brain functions; it can cause headaches, affect your concentration and mood, and can even lead to increased feelings of stress and anxiety. Our brains cannot function properly without water because it's necessary for so many cellular functions and metabolic processes. Water helps to increase blood flow and oxygen to your brain while boosting cognition and concentration. You need to be drinking at least two liters of water every day to keep your mind healthy—this is not counting sodas, teas, or coffee, it needs to be pure water. Another drink that can help your cognitive function is caffeine. While it does hurt some people's sleeping patterns, it has been shown in studies that consuming coffee in the morning can help to boost cognitive function and lower the risk of developing several cognitive disorders.

Specific Foods that Aid the Brain

While balance is important in your diet when fueling the brain, certain foods have components that specifically boost the health of our minds. This doesn't mean that you should eat only these foods and you'll be fine. Your diet needs to be balanced, but focusing on these foods will help to boost your cognitive functioning and support your quest to declutter.

There's a reason your mother always told you that it was important to eat your greens! Green, leafy vegetables such as kale, broccoli, and spinach, contain compounds known as glucosinolates that prevent oxidative stress, protect your cells and therefore prevent the risk of developing neurodegenerative disorders (Marengo, 2020). In fact, not only the green ones, but all cruciferous vegetables are good for brain health for this reason, such as bok choy, cabbage, cauliflower, and Brussels sprouts.

As previously mentioned, oily fish is also good for brain health because they are a good source of omega-3 fatty acids. In addition to helping to maintain membranes, omega-3 also increases blood flow to the brain leading to better cognition and can be found in most oily fish, such as salmon, tuna, herring, and sardines. Nuts and seeds are also good for the brain because they contain omega-3 as well as antioxidants and vitamin E, both of which help to protect your brain cells from damage. You can eat nuts and seeds as a healthy brain-boosting snack or add them on top of salads for a little extra crunch. Another food group that helps to increase your vitamin E levels is whole grains. This includes brown rice, barley, bulgur wheat, oatmeal, and whole-grain bread. These are easy staples to add to your lunches and dinners that will greatly benefit your mind.

Also praised for their antioxidants and therefore cognitive-boosting abilities are berries. They may be small, but they pack a serious punch in terms of antioxidants such as anthocyanin, catechin, and caffeic acid. Similarly, dark chocolate is a good food to add to your diet because of the many antioxidants it contains. Studies have shown that these potent chemicals improve the communication between cells in your CNS, increase plasticity, and help the cells form new connections which boost memory and concentration (Marengo, 2020). The antioxidants in dark chocolate, or specifically cocoa, are called flavonoids, and they help the growth of blood vessels and neurons. Adding berries and dark chocolate to your diet is important for good brain health and ultimately decluttering your mind. Unfortunately, this isn't a sign to eat a mountain of chocolate each night! But if you're craving a block, it can benefit you to listen to that craving. Both chocolate and berries can be eaten as healthy desserts, or berries can be added to your morning oatmeal or smoothie. Soy products offer another powerful source of antioxidants; more specifically, polyphenols, which help to prevent cognitive decline as we age. This includes soy sauce, soy milk, tofu, tempeh, soybeans, and edamame beans.

Avocado has grown in popularity in the last decade or so, making a regular appearance as a toast topping, and lucky for us, it's good for our brains, too! This is because it's loaded with unsaturated, healthy fats that help with the general functioning of our brains as well as working to lower our blood pressure. This is good for our brains because high blood pressure is the root of several cognitive problems. Other than avocados, there are a few other foods that contain healthy fats such as nuts and seeds. Peanuts are particularly good for the mind, as they contain a high proportion of unsaturated fats as well as vitamin E and resveratrol, which is an antioxidant that protects your neurons and cells.

Lastly, eggs should be a staple of your diet for their part in brain support. An easy breakfast food, they contain a number of different B vitamins as well as folic acid, both of which help your brain to expand and prevent cognitive decline.

Optional Brain-Boosting Supplements

While supplements may seem like a tempting option to get all of the vitamins, minerals, and antioxidants that we have gone through in order to develop some kind of super-brain, this is unnecessary.

If you are eating a balanced diet, with a variety of fruits and vegetables, healthy fatty fish, lean proteins, whole grains, and legumes, there is no need to add supplements. You might consider taking various brain-boosting supplements if you have health conditions that cause deficiencies, or if you have a diet that prevents you from eating certain foods. For example, if you cannot eat fish, or choose not to, it's wise to get an omega-3 supplement. However, if you're eating a balanced diet, then taking supplements for vitamins B, C, or E, beta-carotene, or magnesium will only help brain function if you are specifically lacking in them. Otherwise, it will not make much of a difference, except to your wallet.

The Necessity of Movement

Our bodies were created with the intention of movement. Our ancestors spent their days in constant motion, running and sprinting to hunt, walking for miles to gather berries and plants to eat. However, as the world and technology have developed, we don't move nearly as much as our bodies were designed to. We don't walk long distances because we have cars and public transport to take us places instead. We can drive to get our food, even though it's never very far from where we live. And a large proportion of us spend the majority of our days sitting in front of our computers, clicking away at a keyboard.

Our minds and our bodies suffer from our increasingly sedentary lifestyle. We often focus more on the negative effects it has on our bodies, but it's also profoundly harmful to our minds. Regular exercise helps our minds to thrive, to function well, and keeps the flow of goods to the mind consistent. Ensuring that exercise is part of your normal daily routine is an essential part of the balanced lifestyle you need to maintain in order to have a brain that is healthy enough to declutter.

Effect of Exercise on Our Brains

There are several tangible benefits for your mind that you will feel immediately when you begin to exercise, as well as benefits that help you as you age. Exercise has several consequences for our brain. We can create new neurons, increase neuroplasticity (which is essentially how existing neurons adapt and reorganize), and boost the functioning of the neurotransmitters, helping messages to be sent around the brain more easily.

These effects are caused directly by the tendency of exercise to reduce inflammation, reduce insulin resistance, and stimulate the release of the human growth hormone (HGH), which is a chemical that helps to grow new brain cells and blood vessels and repair old ones. Furthermore, while we exercise, there is increased oxygen flow and growth in blood vessels in the area of the brain associated with rational thinking and intellectual performance. There is also an increase in neurotransmitters like serotonin and norepinephrine, which help to increase the speed at which we process information. Regular exercise also increases the levels of chemicals in our CNS that support neurons, called neurotrophins. In these ways, exercise directly increases cognitive functioning, memory ability and general mental health. It can also aid in clearing away brain fog, thereby improving focus and concentration. Exercise allows your mind to be at its peak, and if you are consistently physically active, you will feel the difference in your everyday life, even on days when you don't exercise.

Exercising also has a number of results that benefit your brain indirectly. Exercise has been shown to reduce stress and feelings of anxiety because it reduces cortisol. Cortisol is the stress hormone, and it releases an abundance of endorphins, which increase your general well-being as well as reduce and ease feelings of anxiety and depression. Because exercise reduces stress and decompresses your mind, you also tend to sleep better at night when you are exercising regularly. As we have discussed already, both lack of stress and good-quality sleep are essential for the health of your mind. Because exercise helps with these as well, it's just improving your brain health in another way.

There is no reason not to exercise, and it should be one of the first things you tackle when embarking on your journey to clear your mind from clutter. This doesn't mean that you need to run out and buy a gym membership; there are several easy and accessible ways that you can incorporate exercise into your everyday life that will help you. In fact, one of the best forms of exercise for your mind is brisk walking a few times a week. The CDC recommends getting at least 150 minutes of exercise a week (Centers for Disease Control and Prevention, 2020). While this may sound like a lot, it's just 30 minutes of exercise five days a week. That means you could go for a 30-minute walk for five days of the week and still have two rest days. You can get your heart pumping in many other ways too, and gardening, dancing, or even vigorous cleaning can count as exercise.

Exercises that are Specifically Good for Brain Health

While any kind of movement and physical activity is good for your brain, there are also a number of exercises you can incorporate into your schedule that target specific problems arising from poor brain health and a cluttered mind.

If you struggle with persistent brain fog, you might find that slower and more mindful exercises help to clear it, such as yoga or tai chi. Aerobic classes can also be good for clearing brain fog and helping to improve memory. Other exercises that will help to improve memory can be walking and cycling. Your mind tends to thrive when there is increased blood flow to your brain, and this can be achieved through cardio activities that get your heart rate pumping and your blood flowing. Cardio exercises include running, swimming, walking, cycling, kickboxing, and jumping rope. With an exercise like this, it usually only takes a short amount of time to get a good workout in.

Alternatively, there are exercises that don't leave you sweating but do help your brain in other ways. For example, for those suffering from stress and anxiety, mindful and meditative exercises such as yoga and Pilates can help to ease those feelings. These are great ways to improve your mental health while moving your body. Aerobics and resistance training can also help to alleviate feelings of depression, as they release serotonin, the so-called 'happy' chemical.

You will find that some exercises will benefit you more than others, and you don't have to do them all. Play around and find what works best for you, what fits best into your daily routine, and what makes both your mind and body feel their best.

Making Exercise a Habit

The fact that you should be exercising for your health is probably not a new and groundbreaking idea for you. Most people have known for most of their lives that exercising is essential for your physical health. However, while knowing the benefits exercise provides for the health of your brain might add more motivation, forming a new habit and finding the discipline to exercise regularly and consistently, can be hard when you first start out. But there are several ways to make this easier.

Firstly, ease yourself into it and start small. If you commit to training an hour every day, you're likely to burn out and lose momentum quickly. Start off small and commit to two to three times a week. A little bit is always better than nothing, and if you take your time, you will find it easier to stick to. Then, over time, you can start working out for longer or adding more days until you are up to 150 minutes a week.

Secondly, to form a habit, you need to make it automatic, something that you just have to do in your day, such as brushing your teeth in the morning or having something for dinner. There should be no excuses, it should be instinctive. To make it automatic, you can associate it with triggers. For example, when your alarm goes off, you immediately get into workout gear and head to the door to walk your dog or grab your mat to do a yoga workout. At the end of your workday, change into your workout gear in the bathroom before getting into your car, and head straight to the gym. Trick your brain into being triggered by these things until exercising becomes second nature and a natural part of your everyday routine.

Another way to motivate yourself to exercise is to reward yourself when you manage to be consistent. There are natural rewards that exercising will give you, such as better mental and physical health and improved sleep—but these are long-term benefits that you won't see immediately. Choose to give yourself small, immediate rewards for finishing your workouts, ones that you can only get afterward. They should be small, for example, a favorite coffee or smoothie from a local cafe as you leave the gym, or maybe a hot bath when you get home. Make it something that you would love!

Lastly, start with exercises that you like to do. If you find that walking your dog for 30 minutes is easy and something you enjoy, start with that! You can dance if you find it fun, or any number of activities, as long as your body is moving. If you don't like the routine you have chosen, no amount of willpower will keep you consistent. And consistency is key. Play around with different exercises and routines and see which ones you enjoy the most! The more personalized it is, the better and more effective it will be.

4

What You're Working Toward: The Benefits of Clearing Mental Clutter

I n the previous chapter, we looked at all of the benefits to your brain of living a balanced and healthy lifestyle. However, this is just the first step to decluttering your mind. It is an essential step, though, as you won't be able to declutter your mind if your brain is unhealthy and struggling and your general health is imbalanced. But before we look at those, let's look at the impact of decluttering your mind, and how following through with the rest of this book will improve your life. This is something that has changed my life, and something that will change yours, too.

9 Benefits of Decluttering Your Mind

First and foremost, you will feel a shift in your energy. When your mind is clear, your physical, mental, and creative energy are all ramped up—everything gets a boost, not just your mind. You will find yourself with a greater vitality for life and a renewed sense of passion.

Clearing your mental clutter also helps to lift your brain fog and grants you a certain amount of mental clarity. While it's common to feel fuzzy now and then, you shouldn't go through most of your days like this. Many people don't even realize they are until they start work to clear their minds; suddenly their mind is sharp, and all their thoughts are clear and easily definable. This is what allows you to become more decisive.

Another benefit of decluttering your mind is an increased sense of presence. This is essentially having a "fresh mind." You can move away from conventional thinking, outside of societal ideas of what is important, see things as they truly are, and notice the things that are actually important to you, instead of just seeing what society labels as important.

Mental clarity also helps us to see the details of the world around us and of situations we find ourselves in. This is because our senses are boosted and made clearer. We become more in tune with the smaller details.

Related to this is the added benefit of boosted creativity. Our senses are more tuned to everything; ideas come to you more easily because they have the space to grow in your mind, and your brain is healthy enough that it can think in new and imaginative ways.

Mental clarity also better enables us to see beauty—in ourselves, in our environment, in the people around us, and our daily experiences in general. It allows us to see the 'magic' in our lives, the wonderful in the mundane.

The next benefit of decluttering your mind is the boost it will give your ability to focus and to learn new things. Your mind will expand and take in new information, and you will be able to fine-tune your skills, craft, and talent. With a clearer mind, we also develop an increased sense of flow; everything comes easily and connects, and our minds can find rhythm in how we think and process. This is because there is no more clutter to get stuck on, and your thought process isn't subject to stops and starts.

One of the biggest benefits you will find from decluttering your mind is success. This is more of an indirect benefit, but as you work through decluttering your mind, you will find it easier to prioritize what you need to do to get where you want to be as well as increased motivation and ability to get those things done. Reduced mental clutter allows you to stop being lost, so although you may still have occasional doubts, they will not hold you back anymore. Instead, you will be able to push past your worries and realize that you are capable and that everything you want is possible. Your mind becomes yours to control and direct, and you, therefore, find it far easier to find direction in your life and follow it through. This is how you find success.

Lastly, a lack of mental clutter in your mind also gives you a greater sense of fulfillment and contentment. When our minds are cluttered and busy, we tend to feel stress constantly, but especially when we're sitting still. We struggle to spend quiet time alone because we feel as if there's something we should be doing, something we're forgetting, or something big that we're missing out on. Once we clear the rubbish from our minds, we can sit still without feeling this. We feel more fulfillment from our everyday life, from the small mundane things in our lives, and we can feel content.

Starting the Process of Decluttering

As you can see, the benefits of learning to declutter your mind are extensive and far-reaching. While this can be a complicated process, I've broken it down into 10 simple strategies that you can incorporate into your life one by one. Through this, you will ease change into your life, and slowly feel the clutter in your mind start to clear. Before we begin though, there are a few things you should be aware of as we go through this process. These are not strategies, as such, but rather ways to reframe your thinking as you start to work through the process.

First, you need to practice a degree of mindfulness when starting this method. So often we let thoughts rush through our mind unchecked, and it can be hard to sort through them, or even notice them sometimes. As you start, take moments here and there to stop and witness the thoughts that are going through your mind. In order to filter through your thoughts, you first need to understand what they are.

Next, you need to learn to distinguish between what is part of an intentional life and what isn't. You need to sit down and think about your goals—where do you want to be in five years? Who matters to you? What values are important to you? What does a meaningful life look like to you? You then need to look at how you are currently living, what your short-term goals are, and question whether or not the things you are doing now are going to lead you to the life that you want to have. If they are not, stop doing them. This is how you create an intentional life.

Next, you need to start sitting with emotions. That might sound uncomfortable, or even frightening, but it's important. Similar to our thoughts, we can often feel overwhelmed by emotions but be unable to actually identify them or where they stem from. We avoid negative emotions like anxiety and stress because they scare us. But when we deflect them, we don't actually deal with them; they never go away, and that adds to our clutter. For each of the upcoming strategies to be fully effective, you will need to learn how to confront your emotions. After you've sorted through them, you will have a clearer vision of those that are helping you and those that are not, and this will enable you to eliminate the ones that are holding you back. You need to do the same with your thoughts—being able to identify them also helps you to pinpoint the ones that bring you down.

Finally, you need to let go of expectations. While it's important to have goals and a view of what you want your life to be, we shouldn't let these ideas completely control us. Life is unpredictable, and things may—and frequently do—go differently than we planned, but that doesn't necessarily mean it's not good for us. Letting go of expectations is not about settling for less or letting people hurt us. It's about recognizing that we cannot predict everything, we cannot control everything, and we need to let go of the idea that life should be perfect.

These are essential practices to keep in mind as we move through this book. They should form the basis of everything we do, and you should always be conscious of them as we work through the different strategies. Now that I have laid the foundation for you to declutter your mind, let's start looking at the concrete ways that we are going to make that happen.

5

Strategy #1: Declutter Your Physical Space to Declutter Your Mental Space

The first strategy we're going to look at is the importance of decluttering your physical space to declutter your mental space. While it might seem odd to start this journey outside of your mind instead of with something internal, you cannot achieve mental clarity if your physical space is crowded or chaotic.

When we first think of clutter, we often imagine the house of a hoarder, filled to the ceiling with rubbish and useless things. But it doesn't have to be that dramatic to have a negative effect. Still, most of us have more clutter than we recognize, and it's far more destructive to our physiological health than we realize. Physical clutter can be anything and everything, from countertops that are constantly filled with items we haven't yet thrown away, to clothes that pile up in our bedroom, to bathroom counters filled with products, or tables covered in papers, empty cups, and other litter. Think about your closet, for example. How many of your clothes do you actually wear? If you're like most people, then you're likely to wear the same five outfits on repeat and ignore the remaining 60% of clothes in your closet. Yet, the next time we're at the mall, we'll pick up something new to add, even if we don't need it! We spend all our money just filling our lives and our homes with things, and because we can't possibly use all of it, it's just clutter.

Clutter doesn't live only in our physical space, either. As our world moves online more and more, so does our clutter. Our phones are filled with thousands of notifications from our apps, text messages and emails. We have numerous social media applications where we communicate to the same group of people, just in slightly different ways. We clutter our social lives too, filling our calendars to the covers so that we have no time to breathe for ourselves.

All of this is physical clutter, and it contributes to our psychological struggle and mental clutter because it creates and builds stagnant energy within us, making us restless. So, we need to tackle this first before anything else.

Why We Have Physical Clutter

More often than not, physical clutter is the symptom of another problem, often emotional or mental. There is always an underlying reason why we choose to fill our lives with more things or hang onto them far longer than they are useful. Understanding why we clutter our lives is the first step in learning to declutter.

Sometimes, we hang on to something because of the memories we have attached to it. Perhaps you have a dress that you used to love wearing 10 years ago. You wore it on some vacations that you remember fondly, and it reminds you of a time in your life that you loved. But it doesn't fit you, it hasn't fit for a few years, and it probably won't fit again anytime soon. It, therefore, has no purpose for you and has become clutter. But you keep it because looking at it reminds you of a lot of good times, and some part of you feels that letting go of it will erase those memories.

Similarly, we often keep things because we have an emotional attachment to them. We often do this with childhood objects, but we can also do it with possessions from when we are adults, too. Many of us keep the stuffed toy we had as a child for far longer than we should because it provides a sense of comfort for us. It's familiar and reminds us of home and a more simple, fun time. So, we keep it long past when it's scruffy and falling apart.

Another reason we clutter is through a sense of obligation or guilt. Have you ever been given a gift that you didn't quite like or have a use for? Something that wasn't quite you? Do you still have it? Maybe grandma knitted you a hideous neon yellow sweater four Christmases ago, and even though you immediately knew you would never be caught dead in it, you also knew that she put a lot of time and effort into it, and you couldn't bring yourself to throw it away. We tend to clutter our homes with things we are given because of feelings of guilt and obligation, even when we know we'll never use them.

The last reason that we clutter is a lack of impulse control. Some people struggle with this more than others, but I'm sure we've all had the experience of buying something because it was on sale, and when we got home we realized we didn't really want it all that much. This is made worse by the prevalence of online shopping— you just need to open up your laptop, and with a few clicks you can get a whole new wardrobe delivered! However, impulse buys are hardly ever items that we need, and more often than not, they just add to the pile of things already sitting in our cupboards that we are not actively using.

There are always reasons behind why we gather clutter and collect more things than we could ever need. You need to look at these reasons and try and determine which ones explain why you collect clutter. Understanding why you do this and confronting it is the only way to stop.

What Your Clutter Says About You

How do you start to identify why you're collecting stuff in the first place? While it can help to have a clear-out of your physical clutter, if you haven't solved the root of the problem you'll continue to add more things, and your life without clutter won't last for very long. We have to treat the cause before anything else; otherwise, you will always have a problem.

First, you need to identify the objects in your home that would be classified as clutter. These are the things you own that serve no real purpose, stuff you haven't used in months, or possessions that you've never used and never will use. It's those items that don't give you joy to look at, they just exist in your home, either because you feel obligated to keep them or because you can't be bothered to throw them out or give them away.

Go through your home and identify how much of what you own falls within this definition of clutter, and then identify why you bought it or kept it in the first place. Was it a sense of obligation or emotional attachment? Was it an impulse buy that you've regretted ever since? Figure out which of these reasons directly relate to you and why you have kept these useless items. Once you have figured this out, you will be able to determine the mental root of your problem. If you hang onto things because of emotional attachment, you might find that it's linked to problems you have of letting go generally. You will probably also find that your mental clutter issues are linked to this too; perhaps it manifests as anxiety and stress, and you fret specifically about what you should have done or choices you should have made, and you struggle to let go of the little things. If the cause of your clutter is impulse buying, maybe this is because you don't think through the long-term consequences of decisions or because you're struggling emotionally and you rely on the brief boost of serotonin that impulse buying gives you. If you hold onto things because of the memories they hold, maybe you have problems with moving on and separation anxiety, and keeping physical things helps you to feel connected to people or places that you have lost.

Physical clutter becomes the signpost for your mental clutter, and it tells us what you are struggling with psychologically. Understanding the psychological roots of your actions is the first step to solving them.

The Effects of Clutter on Your Physical Well-Being

While we may think of our minds and our physical spaces as two separate things, they are heavily intertwined. They're both a reflection of one another, and each has the ability to affect the other. There is a strong correlation between the physical clutter a person may have and the mental clutter. It has been shown not only that physical clutter can negatively affect your mind and your general well-being, but also that the reasons for your physical and mental clutter are often linked.

There have been several studies on the link between your physical space and your mental well-being. Research by the University of New Mexico examined how clutter changed our attachments to our home, and it was found that because people identify with their homes and find comfort and peace there, the amount of clutter one accumulates can interfere with that feeling of peace (Roster et al., 2016). This study found that people who accumulate clutter tend to see their homes as a physical extension of themselves and their worth. They tend to fill their homes with things to appease a certain distressing feeling within themselves, and it becomes an act of comfort. However, as their homes become more and more cluttered, it tends to exacerbate their negative feelings, as they become trapped in a space that is dysfunctional and stressful. Essentially, we start to collect clutter because our mental space is overwhelmed and cluttered, and the physical clutter, in turn, just augments this problem.

One of the biggest impacts physical clutter can have on you is to reduce your general sense of well-being. Your home should be a retreat from the stresses of the world, and it should bring you peace. When it's full of clutter and becomes hard to move around in, it causes you more stress, and it becomes your enemy. It is another thing that you have to struggle with and sort out, rather than being the place that allows you to get away from any type of struggle. This causes a constant stress that isn't alleviated, and stress to that extent breaks down your mental and physical health.

Cluttered spaces also tend to lead to unhealthy decisions when it comes to food. I think we've all been in the situation where a kitchen that is cluttered and full of dirty dishes puts us off making dinner, causing us to reach for the takeout menu instead. Studies investigating this suggest that it's because clutter stresses us out and makes us feel out of control (Vartanian et al., 2016). Clutter, therefore, causes us to more easily reach for snacks and unhealthier options.

As these studies show, the chaos in your home caused by clutter can also have a significant impact on our mental health and cause underlying issues to be worsened. Physical clutter causes stress in general, and if you're suffering from chronic stress or mood disorders such as anxiety or depression, existing in a cluttered space is going to make that worse.

Strategies for Physical Decluttering

As with everything in life, it seems, decluttering your physical space is easier said than done. If you just go in, guns blazing, you're unlikely to get very far. Just like you need strategies to mentally declutter, it is important to have strategies to physically declutter too.

Set a Timeline and Goals

One of the first things you need to do when tackling your physical clutter is to create a plan. If the physical clutter in your life is an enemy, the best way to defeat is to create a comprehensive plan of attack. To do this, you're going to set out your goals for what you want to accomplish and create a timeline for how long you want it to take. Starting with specific goals and a plan reduces frustration and confusion because it allows you to know exactly what you're doing and when you're doing it.

To start off, write down or create a map of all the rooms, or smaller areas, that you would like to declutter. Create a scale of the level of clutter, for example, 1-5, with 1 being relatively easy while 5 is extraordinarily messy and chaotic. Assign a level to each of the areas and then based on this, you can roughly estimate how long each area will take. From this estimate, create a timeline for your project. Assign each room a date that you would like to complete it by. Don't overload yourself—tackle one area or room at a time, and give yourself more time than you think you'll need for each space, as well as for the whole process in general. This isn't something you should race through; you should take your time. It's not about finishing first, it's about doing the best job.

This timeline will be completely personal and depend on the level of clutter that you have as well as how big your rooms are and how much free time you have. But it's an essential first step.

Creating a Sorting System

When you begin your decluttering process, you're going to do it a certain way; you're going to create five containers for all the things in that room. It doesn't help to just pick out the things that you don't use anymore; to truly sort through, you need to take out everything. You then sort them into the following boxes:

Put away: These are the items that you're going to keep. They are useful items that you either use in your everyday life or will need regularly. There will be items that you only use seasonally, and you should allow for one or two things that don't have much of a purpose but do have sentimental value. When you have emptied every room into the five boxes, this is the box you'll unpack and return the contents, hopefully in an organized way that flows.

Recycle: Just because you are decluttering your life doesn't mean that it needs to contribute to landfill! Any empty jars or other items that can be recycled should be sorted into this box and then taken to a recycling depot.

Fix: Another variety of clutter is items that have broken that you just haven't got around to fixing yet. Put these in a box, and then over time, work at either fixing them yourself or taking them somewhere to get fixed. Then, you can use them again!

Trash: In this box we're going to put items that have outlived their lifespan. They cannot be recycled or used again, and you cannot use them anymore, so they are going straight into the garbage from this box.

Donate: Just because something is clutter to you doesn't mean that someone else can't use it! Create a pile for all of your items, clothes, dishes, or blankets, that have never been used in your home but could likely be welcomed and used by someone else.

More General Tips for Decluttering Your Life

As you approach this physical decluttering process, there are a few things to keep in mind. First of all, take this one step at a time. The process of clearing out physical clutter can feel overwhelming when you realize how much you have to work through and just how much stuff you actually have. So take small steps and work through it all slowly. If it helps, you can even tackle your room one cupboard or drawer at a time.

It will also help if you can find support from other people who are doing the same thing. Maybe try and encourage someone in your life to declutter their space too, or get your partner to help you with your home. Or you can always find support in online communities. You can also further encourage yourself by taking before and after photos of each goal that you reach, and you will find that seeing the difference so starkly will help motivate you to carry on. Another motivating tip is to make it fun, make a game out of it! Challenge the rest of your house to help out. Maybe you have to find three items you don't use in three minutes, and you can race and see who wins. If you're enjoying the process, it is going to be easier, go quicker, and you're more likely to follow through.

Sentimental items are going to be the hardest to part with. If you have large sentimental collections, like all of your childhood books, for example, remember that a half-done job is better than nothing. Start by just giving away half of what you need to clear out, and you can always do the rest later. Give your heart time to adjust. You can also essentially quarantine items that you're not sure about giving away—put them in a box and hide them away for a set period, like six months. If you don't use them at that time, or even think about them, then you can feel better about getting rid of them.

Most importantly, be kind to yourself. Depending on why you hang onto things, certain items will be harder than others to get rid of. Maybe it's those that have memories or emotions attached. As long as you're sending more things out of your home than you're bringing in, you are decluttering. It can be as long a process as you need.

Strategy Summary: Declutter Your Home

You cannot find mental peace and space if you're living in physical chaos. Physical clutter creates stress and adds to mental clutter, so it needs to be the first thing to go when we start to declutter our minds. Do this by methodically going through your home and clearing out using categories, a timeline, and goals.

6

Strategy #2: Breathing and Meditation

Meditation and mindfulness are key practices that can help you clear your mind of clutter and chaotic thoughts and help you to regain control over your mind. These are calming practices that are highly beneficial for your mental health and everyday happiness.

What Is Meditation and How Can It Change Your Brain?

Meditation is essentially a practice in which you're aiming to reach a state of heightened awareness and focus. It's a technique whereby you empty your mind to reach a complete state of calm and is basically an exercise in changing your consciousness and how you perceive the world and yourself.

The benefits of meditation are rooted in the fact that it can physically morph your brain, as well as the way that you think. To some extent, it prevents our brain from decaying as we age, as it helps to preserve the grey matter of our brain. While this is a benefit that you will only feel later in life, meditation has also been shown to increase the volume of certain areas of your brain, which can completely change the way you think and process. For example, the hippocampus, which controls memory, learning, and emotional regulation, tends to increase in size as a result of meditation. On the other hand, meditation causes the amygdala to shrink over time, and this is the gland that produces feelings of fear, stress, and anxiety (Walton, 2019). As these areas change, so does how we feel, and this helps us to improve our mood, general well-being, and cognitive functioning.

Overall, the act of meditation improves concentration and attention, which can help to offset the chaotic nature of mental clutter by allowing you to take back control of your mind. Every time you meditate you are reclaiming your attention and directing it where you want it to be, thereby training yourself to block out everything else in the process. Like a muscle, the more you practice and train it, the better you become. Studies have shown that just a few weeks of meditation can increase your concentration by an impressive 16% (Walton, 2019).

Lastly, meditation has been shown to be an effective treatment for mood disorders such as anxiety and depression and has proven to generally reduce the effects of daily stress. This is largely because it helps you to quiet the negative thoughts and emotions that can rule your mind, especially when you're suffering from a mood disorder. It also creates the space for you to practice moments of peace that allow you to breathe and get some perspective. Studies involving thousands of patients have shown that continual meditation practice over several weeks can greatly help reduce symptoms of anxiety and depression (Goyal et al., 2014). If you are someone that finds yourself constantly overwhelmed, meditation can help to ease the struggle of daily life.

Types of Meditation

What do you think of when you hear the word meditation?

Is it a hippie sitting cross-legged with their eyes closed, breathing deeply and humming softly to themselves? Some variation of that?

While this is how many of us picture meditation, it's only one way of many that you can practice it. Meditation is a highly personal activity, as it's about sitting and spending time in your own mind. Therefore, different people will respond better to different types of meditative practice. If you find that you struggle to sit down and be still, then forms of meditation that use movement might be more suitable for you. If you need to be still to be calm, still forms of meditation will probably work best for you. The key is to try a few out and see which feels best for you. So, let me take you through the most popular variations.

Concentration Meditation

This is foundational meditation that most of the other types are built from. It's a popular practice and concerned with connecting to and quieting your mind to create a deep focus. You can do it either guided, with someone talking you through it, or unguided.

Heart-Centered Meditation

This type of meditation shifts the focus from your head to your heart. You start by quieting your mind and then spending your practice focusing on your heart, the energy in the middle of your chest.

Mindfulness Meditation

This form of meditation is about taking a step back and being observant of how your mind works and where the negativity in your mind is focused. It teaches you to observe your negative thoughts without giving in to them and trains you to simply let them pass through and out of your mind again.

Tai Chi or Qigong

If sitting still makes you feel restless, you might be better suited to a moving meditation style like tai chi or qigong. They are both forms that combine physical movements with focus and breathing techniques.

Transcendental Meditation

This style involves taking a mantra, a phrase, word, or sound, and repeating it over and over to create focus, quiet your thoughts, and instill a greater sense of awareness.

Walking Meditation

This style is exactly as it sounds—you meditate as you walk, concentrating on all the physical elements that make up walking. It's a method to quiet your mind and your body, and you will often find your breathing starts to match to your footsteps.

How to Practice Meditation

Meditation is a simple and accessible practice that doesn't require anything but yourself and a quiet room. Set aside time each day to meditate, and in the beginning, it's especially important to meditate at the same time every day. This should be a slot when you're not in a rush to get anywhere, so if you don't have a lot of time in the morning, choose instead to meditate in the evening. When you start, don't aim to do it for longer than 5-10 minutes. It will be difficult to go longer than that at first, you need to build up to it. Every day you do it, you can add more time as it becomes easier. To create the right environment, you can dim the lights and light some candles, or even incense.

If you are doing a still form of meditation, choose a place to sit or even lie, if you find that more comfortable. However you have positioned yourself, it needs to be comfortable enough that you can sit like that without fidgeting for an extended period of time, but not so comfortable that you fall asleep! Keep your hands on your legs or your stomach if you are lying down. You then need to start breathing deeply and close your eyes, lower your gaze, or focus on a predetermined object. Breathe slowly and deeply, focusing on your breath and trying to funnel quiet into your heart and mind.

Meditation is not something that comes naturally to most people. However, the more that you do it, the easier it will become. You will find it easier to slip in and out of a meditative state and will find it easier to meditate for longer. While there is a temptation when you start to practice meditation to suppress your emotions to feel calm, this is not helping you to achieve a true meditative state. Instead, allow your emotions to arise, but step back from them and observe. The goal is not to clear your mind completely, it's natural for your thoughts to wander. Instead, acknowledge these thoughts, then let them go and return your focus to your breathing.

Guided Meditation

If you continue to struggle in the beginning, many people prefer to start and persist with guided meditation instead. This is where you listen to an audio recording of a narrator guiding you through your meditation. Depending on the narrator, this can consist of creating an intention for the meditation, guiding you through making yourself comfortable, creating mental imagery, or guiding your breathing. A guide helps you to cultivate mindfulness and find support in your beginning practices. You just pop in your headphones, set a time, and the guide helps you with the rest.

To practice guided meditation, there are many places that you can go to find resources. There are free meditation apps, such as InsightTimer, that offer over 700,000 guided meditations as well as an opportunity to connect with others who are also meditating. Some websites offer free guided meditations, such as UCLA Mindful, Mindfulness Exercises, Smiling Mind, and the University of California, San Diego Center for Mindfulness. Additionally, there are YouTube channels that provide music and images for a meditative state.

If you want a more in-depth collection of meditations, you can also purchase an app or use one that has a subscription. Applications such as Headspace have guided meditations for everything from insomnia to work-related stress, and even also have workouts designed for your body and your mind! Paid apps like Calm are full of guided meditations designed to help you to fall asleep, while YogiApproved has meditation, yoga, and fitness videos available. Sattva and Chopra are excellent apps that link more to the spirituality of meditation.

Whatever you need, there is an application for you, so just pop in your earphones and try it out!

Breathing Techniques and Why They Work

When you're practicing meditation, breathing plays an essential role in helping to center and calm you. Even when you're not meditating, though, learning proper breathing techniques as well as calming ones are essential for learning to bring your body back under your control.

How do you breathe when you're feeling stressed or anxious? Short and shallow breaths, right? This is because your heart is racing, and your lungs just can't keep up. However, when you focus on breathing slowly and deeply, you can reverse this feeling of panic. It can clear your mind and help you to focus again.

We don't often think about our breathing that much—and why would we? It's something that we do automatically. But with a few techniques, we can use our breathing to enable oxygen to flow better around our body and our brain, calming our nerves, and reducing negative feelings; it can even help to improve your attention span and lessen any pain that you may have. Mastering different breathing techniques can also help to foster happiness and allow us to regulate any negative impulses we may have. Studies have shown that practicing proper breathing techniques can even help to curb addictive behavior such as smoking and drinking (Legg, 2018).

Breathing deeply and more mindfully outside of meditation is a wonderful way to calm and nourish your mind and your body. It is one of the best things you can do to give yourself mental clarity.

Different Breathing Techniques

There are several different specific breathing techniques that you can practice that can help you reap all of the benefits that have just been mentioned. Different breathing techniques work well for different situations. Some will help you to wake up and feel more alert, while others are better suited to help you calm down to fall asleep. You can play around with them and try a few different ones to see which ones work for you.

Equal Breathing

Equal breathing is a technique that you could consider incorporating into your nighttime routine, as focusing on your breaths can help calm racing thoughts and prepare your mind for sleep:

You can be lying or sitting or really in any position for this technique. Closing your eyes can help if you are trying to fall asleep.

Through your nose, inhale for 4 counts, and then exhale for 4 counts.

Do this over and over, and once you get the hang of it, you can increase your inhalations and exhalations to 6 or 8 counts.

Abdominal Breathing Technique

When you find yourself overwhelmed by stress before a big presentation or meeting, abdominal breathing is the way to go. When you are stressed, it can be really hard to control your breathing, so it might be a struggle at first. But, by slowing your breaths, you slow your heart rate, and your stress will slowly settle, as it's physically impossible to panic when you are breathing slowly and deeply into your abdomen. Practicing this regularly every day can even help reduce blood pressure and your resting heart rate:

Place one hand on your heart and one hand on your belly.

Take a deep breath in through your nose, and focus on filling your diaphragm so that you feel a slight stretch in your lungs. It might help to imagine you're breathing into your stomach.

Do this for 10 minutes, taking 6-10 slow deep breaths each minute.

Progressive Muscle Relaxation

When we're feeling stress, our body reacts by seizing and bunching up as our muscles contract. This breathing technique is perfect to counteract that contraction. You can do this anywhere, from your office chair to your car, and it can help the stresses of everyday life melt out of your body with each passing breath:

Lie down with your eyes closed.

Starting with your toes and moving up, focus on tensing and then relaxing each muscle group for 2-3 seconds.

Begin with your toes, then your feet, your calves and your knees, etc.

Maintain slow and deep breaths the entire time.

You can also do this by timing your breaths with your muscle movements; inhale and hold for 5 counts, tensing the muscles the whole time, and then breathe out your mouth, releasing the tension slowly.

Alternate Nostril Breathing

Are you feeling anxious and run down? Alternate nostril breathing is a good technique to refocus and re-energize yourself, giving yourself the same kick as a cup of coffee would:

Find a comfortable meditative seat.

With your dominant hand, extend your thumb, ring finger, and pinky finger and tuck your middle and pointer finger into your palm.

Press your thumb on the outside of your one nostril. Inhale deeply through the other open nostril, and at the height of your inhalation, take your thumb off and use your ring finger to press your other nostril closed.

Exhale through the open nostril.

Repeat this over and over for 1-2 minutes, ensuring that you are inhaling and exhaling equally with each nostril.

Ocean Breath

This breathing exercise is intended to cleanse you, just as the salty freshness of ocean water would. It's ideal for dissolving negative emotions such as anger or frustration, as it settles and refreshes your mind.

Start by simply inhaling deeper than you normally would.

When you exhale, breathe out through your mouth while constricting your throat muscle. This should cause your breath to sound like waves in the ocean.

Box Breathing

Box breathing is a simple technique that aims to return your breathing to its normal rhythm and can be highly beneficial when you're feeling anxious or highly strung. It's simple and can be done anywhere:

Close your eyes. Inhale slowly to the count of 4 while you focus on the air filling your lungs.

Hold your breath for 4 counts, but don't clamp your mouth or nose shut.

Then, exhale slowly to the count of 4. Repeat for a few minutes, or until calm returns. You can extend the count to 5 or 6 seconds as you go along.

Strategy Summary: The Necessity of Mindfulness

Practices such as meditation and breathing techniques are essential for sweeping clutter from our minds, as it is a practice that actively teaches us how to clear our thoughts, take back control, and let go of negative feelings and emotions. It's a simple and accessible practice you can fit into your everyday life, and it's an integral step in your journal to clarity and peace.

7

Strategy #3: Write Away Your Thoughts

The saying, "It's better out than in," is never more apt than when we speak about negative emotions. Making a practice of writing out feelings and overwhelming emotions greatly reduces our mental clutter, as it allows us to take the junk out of our heads and place it somewhere else—on a piece of paper.

Most of the time, our psyches become cluttered with negative emotions because we ignore them, and we don't sort through them or understand where they're coming from. Through journaling, writing lists, and brain dumping, you can not only get rid of these emotions, but also understand them so that they don't linger or continue to be overwhelming.

Journaling

Journaling is a helpful tool for processing your feelings, thereby helping to reduce stress and anxiety. It is essentially where you just write, possibly in a notebook, and take everything that you are thinking about and splash it out on a page.

Benefits of Journaling

Journaling has plenty of scientifically proven benefits, especially for reducing stress and mental clutter. Most importantly for us, it helps to clear your mind. Just as we declutter our physical space by putting everything into boxes to create a sense of order, journaling allows us to do that for our minds. It allows you to create a sense of order within your thoughts, and even just the semblance of order can greatly help to reduce stress and anxiety.

And as we already know, having a clear mind comes with a myriad of benefits.

Journaling can help you to fall asleep, as you have taken all of your racing thoughts out of your head and put them on paper. It can also improve your memory, both by creating space in your mind and also simply through the act of chronicling your life every day. When you write something down by hand, your brain processes it better and is more likely to commit it to memory. It also helps to boost your health because you are sleeping better and also because you are focusing on your positive feelings and reducing your stress levels, both of which vastly benefit your physical health.

Journaling is great not only because it boosts mental clarity, but it also has a few direct benefits, such as being able to track your emotions, reach goals, and reduce mood disorders such as anxiety and depression. All of these indirectly help you to clear mental clutter, too.

Tracking emotions is an excellent tool for your mental health; it not only helps you to process your emotions, but it also allows you to find patterns in your moods. It becomes easier to identify what triggers negative emotions and what triggers positive ones, so you can chase the positive events and try to avoid or reduce the influence of the negative ones in your life. This alleviates the effects of anxiety or depression, as it helps to uncover the root of these problems, giving you something to actively work through.

By using this technique, you can find your goals more reachable. This is partly because working through your feelings will help you to clearly see them, but also because writing out what you want holds you accountable. It solidifies your goals in your mind, which makes you more likely to look for opportunities that will lead to them and also gives you the space to work through the small steps you need to take to reach them.

The key to feeling the effects of journaling is to be consistent; it's something you need to do every day. Essentially, five minutes is all you need. It's easy to create a habit of doing something every day when it only requires five minutes, just make it part of your routine. Add it to the mental list of things you need to do in the morning before you leave—brush teeth, wash your face, eat breakfast, journal. This will help you persevere with it.

Different Types of Journaling

There are several different journaling types you can try, and each is good for different things. Like most things in life, the type that works for you will depend on your personal preference.

Stream of Consciousness Journaling

This type of journaling is essentially just writing—write whatever is on your mind without editing and without stopping, and just letting all the anxious thoughts flow out of your mind. It allows you to notice what you're thinking. However, if you have a restless mind prone to racing thoughts, you might find it hard to do this and complete a single thought before the next one jumps in.

While exercising this style, it's important to refrain from judging and editing yourself, and instead, just let the thoughts flow. Don't try to be meaningful, and just follow your thoughts down the rabbit holes they may lead to—that's how you get to the root of things.

Journal Prompts

If looking at a blank page and wondering where to start makes you feel anxious or overwhelmed, journal prompts might be the way to go. This can also be helpful if you have an abundance of thoughts racing through your mind and need to concentrate on just one. Prompts are questions that help you to reflect on a single feeling, emotion, or thought at a time.

You can find prompts in many ways; simply Google "journal prompts" or download apps that give you different prompts every day. Some examples are Five Minute Journal, Day One, and Memento. When using journal prompts, aim to be honest and transparent when answering the prompts, doing otherwise will only hurt yourself.

Bullet Journaling

Bullet journaling is a productive kind of journaling, where you can take all the to-do lists and errands you have bouncing around in your head and put them on paper. Bullet journaling is essentially using a planner, but with a more reflective aspect. You can include a daily to-do list, a calendar and habit trackers; and there are hundreds of templates online for you to explore and test out.

The key to success with this type of journal is writing every day; if you don't, you will begin to feel overwhelmed when you check it every few days and there are piles of things to do and catch up on. It's meant to decrease your stress, not add to it.

Creative Journaling

Finally, we have creative journaling. This is a chance to take a break and let your imagination run wild. Creativity is an innate human quality, and while you might think you are not even remotely creative, this type of journaling can help you to exercise that muscle and find it again.

You can do anything when you creatively journal. You can write stories, draw, scrapbook, paint, or cover a book with quotes. Take a blank journal and go wild, follow your inclinations and imagination and see where it takes you. It will become a form of self-care, as you express yourself through something that brings you joy.

Writing Lists

One of the biggest things that clutter our heads is the sum total of all the things we need to do. We are living these fast-paced lives, juggling everyday errands with demanding jobs and familial and social responsibility—and our brains are constantly throwing all these to-dos around to make sure we don't forget any of this.

It's exhausting!

While it may seem like a simple solution, writing lists can be a great way to ease this stress from your mind. It's easier for your memory, as even the act of writing things out can help you to remember them. It takes things that are abstract and almost intangible, such as goals and aims, and makes them concrete, which makes them accessible and easier to work toward. This in turn helps you to be increasingly goal-orientated, more productive, and achieve more. Even if you don't complete your list for a day, you probably got far more done than you would have if you weren't working from a list.

Most importantly, writing lists is a crucial aspect of decluttering your mind and easing chronic stress, as it creates order in your day and makes everything feel more manageable. This allows you to be productive without feeling overwhelmed. Your brain is sort of trained to be productive, and anytime you can check something off, you get a small sense of accomplishment! This is an excellent tool for reducing the daily chaos that fills your mind as well as encouraging productivity and accomplishment.

Helpful Tips for Writing a To-Do List

Writing a to-do list is an easy task and undoubtedly something you have done before. The only difference is that now we're going to make a habit out of it. You can do this in any planner, blank journal, or even your bullet journal. Create a new to-do list each day. It doesn't matter if you don't finish the to-do list, anything left can be transferred to the next day, but try and be realistic with what you can do in a day.

There are a couple of rules you should stick to when compiling a to-do list. First and foremost, keep the tasks a manageable size. For example, if you're doing an assignment for work, break it down into chunks. So instead of writing "finish assignment" on the to-do list, write "research for assignment," and "outline assignment." The trick is to break big tasks down into smaller steps. This feels so much more manageable and allows you to tick off more as you go along, creating a greater sense of accomplishment.

It's also important to prioritize your to-do list, putting the more pressing tasks first and then going down in order or importance. You could even color code your list, writing the important errands in red and the ones that have more flexibility in green. Another tip is to add dates for when you want something to be done. This is a great technique to allow you to easily transfer it into a calendar so that you can see your month at a glance. This isn't only very satisfying and calming, but it also helps you to better prioritize your everyday to-do list.

The rest is a personal preference. You can make more than one list for every day, such as one for household errands and the other for work. You can structure it in different ways, it all just depends on what works well for you, and what makes you feel both organized and productive.

Strategy Summary: Physically Rid Yourself of Toxicity

Getting your thoughts, emotions, and worries out on paper in the form of anything from journaling to brain dumping, is a brilliant way to declutter your mind. It helps to order your thoughts and is almost a physical act of removing excessive thoughts from your mind, allowing for more space. This helps you to focus, feel calmer and curb emotional disorders such as anxiety and depression.

8

Strategy #4: Stop Multitasking

As a society, we tend to praise busy people. People that seem like they're handling a thousand things at once and still thriving despite doing two things at a time and never having a moment to rest. Isn't that the picture of competency and productivity?

In actuality, multitasking is not good for our minds or our body and is a significant contributor to your mental clutter. While we may think that our minds are easily able to flit between numerous tasks, it is actually very taxing physically. Each time we do a small shift, there is a cost to our brain; and when we do this multiple times in the space of a few minutes, we are causing significant damage that can lead to permanent brain damage (Oshin, 2018). This damage has a cumulative effect on the way our brain operates. Over time, multitasking depletes our cognitive processing and reduces our ability to concentrate for long periods of time as our minds get so used to switching between multiple things quickly and become easily distracted.

Furthermore, the more we multitask, the more we burden and overwhelm our minds. This is a significant contributor to mental clutter, as it lessens the abilities of our minds to be still and quiet.

It increases our cortisol levels, causing stress, as well as creating mental fatigue which leads to feelings of anxiety. Over time, you'll begin to feel burnt out, as you are literally depleting the nutrients in your brain. It kills your ability to be creative and kills your impulse control, which can result in bad decision-making. Multitasking is one of the worst things we can do for our minds in so many ways.

These days, our attachment to our devices has made multitasking even more commonplace. How often are you on your phone while doing other things? Replying to emails and texts while working on other things? Scrolling through your Instagram while watching a movie or watching a YouTube video while doing household tasks? Now more than ever, we are subjecting our brains to multiple tasks at once, and the damage it's doing is literally killing them.

Benefits of Focusing on Single Tasks

While there are a multitude of detrimental effects to multitasking, there are equally as many benefits to shifting back and allowing ourselves to take each task one at a time.

It will take a concentrated effort to make this change, and you will need to be determined not to fall back into the multitasking habit. But it's a vitally necessary step in order to undo the damage inflicted by years of multitasking. It's a habit that you have to unlearn, but there are so many positives to choosing to give 100% of your attention to the task in front of you for as long as it needs to get done.

Rebuilds Focus

When we multitask we lose the ability to concentrate for long periods, as our brains are used to switching back and forth constantly. As you start to make a habit of focusing on one task at a time, you will notice that your ability to concentrate increases slowly but surely. Your focus will increase, and this will have a direct, positive effect on your feelings of stress and productivity.

Reduces Feelings of Stress

Multitasking stresses the brain out. It takes more energy, and all the switching back and forth increases the levels of cortisol coursing through our bodies—the stress hormone. In addition, multitasking stresses us out because it reduces our productivity, and simple tasks take far longer than they should.

Focusing on a single task lowers our stress levels because it doesn't release cortisol, so we become more productive when we do one thing at a time. The added benefit is that finishing everything you need to do in a day leaves you with the evening to relax and not spend the whole night stressing about everything you have to catch up on the next day!

More Productive

As we have seen, we are far more productive when we focus on doing one task at a time instead of multiples. Switching always slows us down. In fact, researchers have estimated that taking on more than one task causes us to lose 20% of our overall productivity (McKay, 2020). Imagine all the time we're wasting!

If we spend time on one thing, we inevitably get into a flow, a state of deep focus that allows us you to get more done with much less effort.

Increased Creativity

When your mind is overwhelmed and stressed, it doesn't have the energy to be creative.

When your brain isn't expending all its effort with the multitasking switching, it almost gets restless. But this boredom is positive because it unlocks extra potential by giving your mind time to sit on something, ruminate, and eventually lead to coming up with a new perspective, a new thought pattern, or option it hadn't discovered before.

Focusing on one task boosts your creativity because your brain has time to wander and to deeply focus.

How to Stop Multitasking

As with many activities or routines in our lives, multitasking has become something of a habit for so many of us. It has become hardwired and just a part of how we operate, but you can fight against the compulsion to follow habitual patterns, and there are several small things you can do to help you and your tired brain in that fight. These tips can help you to focus and help to clear the chaos and tension from your mind.

Get Enough Rest and Plan Ahead

Sleep and rest are key for a healthy and well-functioning brain. When you're even slightly sleep-deprived, your ability to concentrate plummets, making it far easier for you to get distracted by the smallest thing. It's critical to get good sleep consistently, though, or you will always struggle to focus on one task at a time. Of course, if you work non-stop throughout the day, even taking tasks one by one, your brain is going to get fatigued, too. The best approach is to take regular breaks throughout the day, get some fresh air or walk around, and let your brain recharge.

Another tip for maintaining focus is to plan your day ahead of time. If you don't have a good idea of how your day is going to go, it's easy to get distracted, lose your direction and end the day without having accomplished much. When you plan ahead, your brain subconsciously prepares for it, and it's easier to focus.

Commit Yourself to the Task

When you constantly allow yourself to be taken away from what you need to do, you are creating a habit of being distracted. In order to commit yourself to what you're doing, it helps if you choose a spot solely for your work, if you learn to say 'no,' and only commit to what you can handle.

The solution to finding your focus is to do your work only at your desk. At our cores, we are creatures of habit; and if we sit at our desks and do online shopping, play games, and distract ourselves as well as doing work, we will create a habit out of it. The key to staying focused on a single task is to condition your brain to associate a certain space with productivity.

Overloading yourself with jobs can also make it impossible to stay focused on a single thing because you are always aware that you don't have time for everything. To stay focused and clear your mind of clutter, you need to find a way to say 'no' when asked to do something that you don't have time for. It's not being rude or unreliable, but rather it's being honest, both with yourself and with others in your life.

Remove All Distractions

Even the strongest psyches will fold under the pressure of relentless distractions—every time our phone pings or an email notification pops up on our computer, our attention is immediately snapped out of focus. It's impossible to keep your concentration on a single task when this happens because as soon as you see it, you start thinking about whatever has been sent to you, and your brain switches straight into multitasking.

So when you sit down to work, put your phone on silent and–even better–in another room. Then turn off notifications on your computer as well to make sure that nothing is going to 'ping' and throw your mind off course!

Strategy Summary: All or Nothing

While multitasking may seem like a tempting way to increase your productivity, it's slowly killing your brain and your productivity. Instead, decrease the time you spend doing multiple things, and focus on completing tasks one at a time. You will find yourself more productive and focused this way, and it's the fundamental code to decluttering your busy mind.

9

Strategy #5: Reframe Your Negative Thought Patterns

Negativity takes up far more space in our minds than positivity does. Think about how you feel when you're experiencing negative emotions such as anger, anxiety, or stress. Overwhelmed? Stuck, even? You probably feel like you have the same thoughts lodged in your head for hours or days, going around in the same circle of negativity. On the other hand, positive emotions tend to be fleeting and light. It might be counterproductive, but the regrettable truth is that we rarely dwell on happiness; it's ours for a moment and then it passes on.

We feel this way because we have a natural negativity bias, which is a tendency for negative emotions to linger and make far more of an impact than positive feelings. Because negative emotions are far heavier and persistent, they make up a lot of our mental clutter in the form of pressure, anxiety, insecurity, and the like. They also make life less enjoyable and detract from our day-to-day happiness. Reversing your negative bias is an important step not only for decluttering your mind, but also for your overall health and happiness.

Negativity Bias and Types of Negativity

The key to ridding your mind of negativity is to try and reverse the negativity bias that we all inherently suffer from. Negativity bias is the tendency to register negative stimuli more readily, as well as to dwell on the events that caused them. It's ingrained in our brains to pick up the tiniest negative stimulus far quicker than they do for positive ones (Cherry, 2019). This psychological discovery explains why traumatic events can linger for decades, why we can recall insults far longer than we can remember compliments, and why we tend to dwell on the bad parts of our day over the good.

While the exact cause of this tendency is unknown, it's likely the result of evolution. As humans, we are designed to be ready to fight for our lives, if necessary; and that ability makes us sensitive to danger and threat. While this may have been a necessary ability for evolution and the success of the human race, in modern life, it's harming us rather than helping us. It affects our relationships, our decision-making skills, and our perception of others. It also damages our relationships with others, as negative actions carry far more weight than positive ones, even if they are smaller and more insignificant, and we automatically expect the worst from people. If we cannot evenly weigh the good and the bad in any given situation, our ability to make decisions is affected because we deeply fear the consequence of any potential negative outcome far more than we desire the positive ones.

Different Types of Negativity

While you may not think that you suffer from negative bias, you inevitably will in some form. Negativity can manifest itself in several different ways:

Filtering: Only noticing the bad in an otherwise positive memory.

Cynicism: A general distrust of people and situations.

Hostility: Instinctive unfriendliness towards others, and an unwillingness to form new friendships and relationships.

Jumping to conclusions: The automatic reaction to assume that something bad is going to happen.

Blaming: The tendency to blame all the negative events in your life on others, to shift responsibility away from yourself, and see yourself consistently as a victim.

Emotional reasoning: Relying on your emotions instead of logic to dictate what is real and valid in your life and what is not.

The fallacy of change: The idea that when things or people change, only then will you be happy. Assuming that your situation is what is making you unhappy.

Catastrophizing: The belief that disaster is inevitable, that nothing ever goes right.

Heaven's reward fallacy: The manifestation of negativity causes you to become bitter or depressed when you have worked hard but things don't go your way, as you are led by the assumption that sacrifice and hard work will always be rewarded.

It's natural to identify with one or more of these manifestations of the negativity bias. It also gives you a good idea of what you're taking on when you are making efforts to undo negative thought patterns and what behaviors and perceptions you need to be cognizant of changing.

Physical Consequences of Negativity

While the consequences to our brains are evident when it comes to negative thinking, there are also substantial effects on our bodies when we allow ourselves to be ruled by negative emotions for extended periods. This is because negative stimuli signal to our bodies that we are in danger, that we are under stress. When we are stressed, our bodies release cortisol, which makes us more alert and focused, prepared to take on any crisis. However, it also puts a lot of pressure on our bodies, and extended periods of this kind of pressure with the consistent releases of cortisol it brings, will start to break down our body.

This can cause many physical problems, such as headaches, fatigue, chest pains, and stomach problems. The breaking down of your body can also affect your mental health, as cortisol disrupts your sleeping patterns and can exacerbate feelings of anxiety and depression. Prolonged negativity can also lead to negative coping mechanisms, such as smoking and drinking.

If you are constantly struggling with your body, feeling tired and worn down regularly, consistent negative emotions could be the underlying cause. Reversing negative thought patterns is vital not only for freeing our consciousness of the clutter it creates, but also for ensuring our best health.

Common Negative Thought Patterns and How to Reverse Them

As there are common manifestations of negativity, there are also common negative thought patterns that we tend to fall into. When we allow these unhelpful perspectives to run rampant, we are letting the clutter that they induce run free, too. To reach a state of mental clarity, you need to identify the negative modes of thinking that you naturally tend towards, and through the tips we will walk through together, reverse them. That's the only way to free your mind of the clutter that negative thinking induces. So, let's look at the most common thought patterns that may be weighing you down.

Black and White Thinking

It is easy to settle on a binary perspective, thinking that something is all or nothing. It's when you believe that someone who isn't altogether good, inherently has to be bad. Or, feeling that you have completely failed at something when one or two things have gone wrong. While we often don't realize it, this is a destructive negative thought pattern. It causes you to give up at a time when, if you just keep pushing, you can still succeed. It causes you to rule out people and situations because you have decided it's not intended for you, when you haven't given them a chance in the first place.

To reverse this point of view, you need to identify when you tend to act or feel this way. You need to acknowledge the grey areas of life, and you need to acknowledge that a few things can go wrong, but that everything can still turn out alright.

Focusing on the Negative

Another negative thought pattern manifests itself in the form of tunnel vision, where the unfavorable is all that you can see. It's natural for us to do this from time to time, to be so weighed down by what has gone wrong that you cannot see the silver lining. However, when this becomes a pattern, it can weigh heavily on your mind with pessimistic clutter.

The only way to reverse the effects of this behavior is to start training yourself to look for the positives, especially in your everyday life. Some practices can help you in this, such as doing gratitude journaling every day, practicing forms of self-care, and meditation. All of these are ways in which you can take a moment and refocus your attention so that you can find small points of happiness. When we are focusing on what we are thankful for instead of everything that's wrong, we inherently feel happier and more fulfilled. It's important to challenge yourself to find the good.

Not Questioning Your Feelings

While all of our emotions are valid, that doesn't mean they're always right. We are often taught to trust our gut instinct, to listen to that little voice inside of our heads, but that voice is frequently guided by negative emotions, fears, anxieties, and a self-defense mechanism. So if we are always listening to that instinct, we can therefore be guided by these detrimental feelings.

To reverse the effects of this, take note when you have a gut feeling, but don't immediately act on it. Try and identify if that instinct is fueled by self-defense or the anxiety that you often experience. Use a journal and tally up the pros and cons of whatever situation you are faced with. By doing this, you can determine whether your intuition is valid, or whether you would be better off following logic instead. Over time, you will be able to correct this thought pattern and instinctively be able to distinguish between hunches that are credible and those that are harmful.

Guilty Thinking

One of the greatest sources of negativity and clutter is based simply on how we think in the language we are unconsciously using. Guilty thinking usually manifests itself in words such as 'have to,' 'should,' and 'must.' It's those thoughts about what we should be doing, what we should have done, and how we should be acting instead of following what we want to do. We tend to be highly critical of ourselves when we don't do what we think we should do.

To reverse this guilt-inducing self-talk, you need to stop using the language. Take time to reflect on what obligations you actually have, how they make you feel, and how to reduce them if they are causing you too many negative emotions. It's also important to be kinder to yourself. It's okay to put your own needs first, before your obligations, and you should not feel any level of guilt about doing so. You would not be harsh with others for putting their own needs first, so you would be wise to extend that same compassion to yourself.

Self-Labeling

Again, this is a need to reevaluate how you think about yourself and how you talk to yourself. Many of us have developed negative language for ourselves without even realizing it. Self-labeling is not always a bad thing, sometimes it can give us a sense of belonging, a sense of identity. However, it becomes negative when we start to call ourselves things like 'loser' or 'failure,' or if we think of ourselves as 'worthless' or in any way 'less than.'

To counteract the critical self-labeling, the first thing to do is be aware that you're doing it. Recognize the way that you talk to yourself, and make a conscious effort to turn that around. Each time you find yourself falling into the harmful self-label habit, switch it to something like a positive statement instead. You can repeat affirmations such as: "I am worthy," "I believe in myself," and "I am doing great." Rewire your thoughts to be positive.

Benefits of Positive Thinking

Negative thought patterns are so bad for your mind and body that you will see improvements merely in their absence. However, purposely moving toward positive thinking also has several benefits for both your mental and physical health.

Having a positive mindset can increase your lifespan. Because it lowers your levels of distress, it also improves your cardiovascular health, decreasing the risk of heart and lung problems as you grow older. It also lowers your level of depression and can help you to better cope during difficult times.

Positive thinking is also a fundamental element of a decluttered and clear mind, preventing negative emotions from lingering and taking up space.

Rewiring Your Brain to Think Positively

The absence of negativity will not automatically switch your thoughts to positivity. While rewiring the negative thought patterns will help, you still have to actively train your brain to start being more positive.

Practices like keeping a gratitude journal are useful because they allow you to take time to be grateful, to stop and recognize all the reasons you have to be positive and happy. Practicing gratitude has been proven to make you healthier and maintain a happier outlook (Emmons 2010). Meditation can also be a good practice to help with this. In general, creating time for yourself and self-care is an important part of living a more positive life. If you are constantly hectic, stressed, and busy with everything else except for yourself, it's hard to recognize all the things in your life that should make you feel positive.

You should also recognize how your negative thoughts manifest, and practice spending time finding the silver linings in bad situations. Learn to be kind to yourself and to practice compassion in how you talk to yourself and how you think about yourself. So much of rewiring your brain to be more positive is about being more mindful and taking note of everything that you have been missing.

Strategy Summary: Reframe Your Mind

Our consciousness has a natural predilection to focus and ruminate on the negative, but doing so destroys our mental and physical health and clutters our minds with feelings of stress, anxiety, and insecurity. To counteract this, you need to reverse your negative thought patterns and actively rewire your brain to think positively. You will find yourself not only happier, but also healthier and more content.

10

Strategy #6: Time for a Digital Detox

Our electronic devices are one of the biggest sources of clutter in our modern world. They are filled with social media apps that we feel we must check throughout the day as well as emails and text apps filled with notifications. Studies have shown that 18% of American adults say that technology is a significant source of stress in their lives, and a study in Sweden found that heavy technology use is linked to poor mental health, sleeping problems, and increased stress (Cherry, 2019). We are compelled to always be available, and the sense of obligation that this creates within us leads straight to pressure and mental clutter that leaves us feeling overwhelmed.

To counteract this, you need a digital detox to clear your mind.

What is a Digital Detox?

A digital detox is when you temporarily disengage from all digital devices for a specific period to reduce stress and cleanse your mind by focusing on being present in the real world. The idea is based on the premise that letting go of online interactions allows you to focus on interacting with people in real life. And without the obligation to be present online, you can focus on the outside world and yourself, which reduces stress.

Signs That You Need to Detox

If you're thinking that your devices don't add to the tension and clutter in your life, you're probably underestimating their power. Our digital life has more of an impact than we usually realize, and a digital detox can benefit everyone. Here are some signs that your electronic devices are becoming a detriment to your everyday health and happiness:

You feel anxious, stressed, or even slightly depressed after spending time on social media.

You cannot go for a few minutes without checking your phone.

You're overly concerned with how many likes, shares, and comments you get on anything that you post.

You're afraid you'll miss something if you are without your phone for a few hours.

The first thing you do when you wake up is go on your phone, and it is the last thing that you do before you fall asleep.

You have trouble doing anything without checking on your phone, whether it is seeing your friends or watching a movie.

Why Should You Do a Digital Detox?

A digital detox is the perfect way to alleviate some of the pressure in your life and allow yourself time to breathe. It will kickstart your mental and physical health and can give you the focus and energy you need on the journey to decluttering your mind.

Because it's such a big part of our everyday lives, we've become blind to how stressful technology is. Reducing your daily tension is one of the most pressing reasons to detox from your devices for a while. A detox can also help to improve your sleep, which is good for both your mental and physical health. Using cell phones, laptops and tablets, especially just before you sleep, can have a devastating effect on your sleep quality. The blue light from electronic devices disrupts our circadian rhythm, and this reduces both how well we sleep and our ability to get to sleep.

Constant device use also makes it particularly difficult to maintain a good work and life balance. For most of us, a lot of our work is conducted on our devices, whether it's on our phones or laptops. When we don't take breaks from our devices, we are also not taking a break from work or the burden that it induces. Furthermore, extensive use of our devices is often linked to mental health problems, such as increased anxiety and depression. This can be exacerbated by the comparison that social media induces because looking at the carefully edited highlights of everyone else's lives can lead to you feeling bad about yourself, or that you're missing out on things you should be doing or that you would like to be doing.

A digital detox helps to remove all of these destructive thoughts from your head and allows you to live in and appreciate your own real life for however long you choose to do it. It can also be beneficial to you to gauge how much time you're wasting online by seeing how much free time you have when you digitally disengage. Once you realize all of the other things that you can do, it may help you to limit your screen time going forward.

Benefits of a Digital Detox

There are abundant benefits that you will gain from a digital detox besides clearing the clutter from your mind. First and foremost, it will give you a lot more free time that you can use to do something constructive that makes you happy. It's estimated that most adults now spend more time on their devices than they do sleeping (Cherry, 2019). Imagine all that time that you've been wasting doing something that has brought you nothing but stress. Detoxing allows you to use that time for something else. You can pick up a new hobby! Maybe try out that sport you have always thought about or spend more time connecting with friends and family in the real world.

A detox can also help you to develop a better sense of mindfulness, particularly when it comes to how long you spend looking at a screen. Once you become aware of what you can do with that time after being away for a while, it will discourage you to scroll mindlessly as you once did. It helps you to reverse the habit of constantly reaching for your device or switching between all your social media apps.

A detox can also specifically provide you with happier and more productive mornings. We have developed the habit of reaching for our phones first thing in the morning, and the moment we click on the first notification, we fall down a rabbit hole that can keep us preoccupied for incalculable minutes—and that sets the tone for your whole day. A detox lets you wake up slowly and naturally, and then you can do what you want. You can read a book, go for a walk, or get a workout done. You can start your day on a much healthier note.

Lastly, and perhaps most importantly, doing a detox will help you to clarify your thoughts and significantly reduce feelings of anxiety and pressure. Being on social media only clutters our minds with broadly useless information and negative thoughts. Taking a break from it gets rid of all that, which in turn, also helps to ease feelings of disquiet and stress. Furthermore, a detox allows you to connect with yourself again, be mindful, and spend time doing things that make you feel good.

How to Do a Digital Detox

A digital detox is something that is best undertaken regularly, especially when we're clearing out the clutter in our heads. The best thing to do is to kick it off with a long detox. First, try a weekend, two or three days where you avoid all of your devices. When you have mastered that, then attempt to do it for a week. If you can, try to stay away from your electronic devices for as long as a month! If you can't manage longer than a few days for work reasons, you could aim for smaller detoxes every day, and commit to not using your devices before and after work.

To start off, make a list of the devices that you use regularly, whether it is daily or weekly. Then, next to each device, list how many hours you spend on it. This will be a complete eye-opener, even if you think that you are fairly conscious of how you spend your time. For most devices, there is an in-built tracker that will tell you your screen time. If, for example, you spend 2.5 hours a day on your phone, that may not seem like a lot on its own. However, 2 hours a day is 14 hours a week; it's 60 hours in a month and 730 hours in a year! That is 30 days–a whole month–spent on your phone in one year; and that's just one of your devices. What you discover as a result of going through this process will shock you and give you a good boost of motivation for a detox.

From here, you can make a list of all the other activities you could do with that time, things you have always wanted to do. Maybe you want to work out more regularly or pick up a new hobby. Then, start to tell people in your life that you are taking time away from your devices. This holds you accountable so that you can't give up after a day or two because you're finding it too much of a struggle. You could also decide on a daily limit for your devices, allowing you to call people and check up on things if you need to.

After you've done that, delete all your social media applications, and block social media sites on your laptop. While you may need to make phone calls, you do not need to scroll through Instagram. Purging your devices of these unnecessary sites will make the detox easier to do.

Strategy Summary: Put Away Your Devices

Technology and all the obligations it carries are a significant source of pressure for many people. Doing a digital detox is essential for cleansing your mind and body of all the toxins that social media and electronic devices induce. It will reduce your stress and anxiety and give you more time to do the things that make you happy and content.

11

Strategy #7: Spend Time in Nature

Have you ever had an intensely stressful day, one where you felt like you could barely breathe, and your mind would not slow down? Then maybe you decided to go for a walk. Something in your restless and overextended heart called you outside, and the minute you stepped into the fresh air, you felt just a little bit lighter.

That's because connecting with the outside world is a natural remedy for a burdened and chaotic mind. Being in nature clears our heads because it reminds us that the world is bigger than our problems and that there are so many beautiful things to be grateful for. Let's dive into how nature can help you on your journey to mental clarity, and how to increase your time outdoors.

How Nature Can Change the Brain

The benefits that nature bestows upon us and our minds are not abstract, it can help to physically change our brain and the way it functions; and taking ourselves outside can have long-lasting, positive effects on our mental health. Studies have shown that living near greener spaces and spending time outside can improve your long-term mental health and that going outside regularly, especially in open green spaces, can radically improve the management of mood disorders. In fact, exposure to nature directly decreases activity in the part of your brain linked to depression, the subgenual prefrontal cortex (Yar & Thorpe, 2020). It has been proven that there is an immediate improvement in mood after being in nature for even an hour, as it allows your mind to clear, and you tend to find it easier to be positive.

Nature is not only good for your spirit, it boosts your general wellness, too. Being in green spaces helps to reduce your heart rate, blood pressure, cholesterol levels, and can improve your sleep. Your body systems begin to calm down when you expose them to nature, reaching for a state of peace. Being outside in natural spaces can also help to improve your memory and cognitive abilities, as even a short exposure to nature has demonstrated improvement to both memory and attention capabilities (Twohig-Bennett & Jones, 2018). Your brain is revitalized when you allow it a moment to empty and to focus on beauty and calm.

However, it's interesting to note that different types of natural spaces have different effects on your body. One type is a wilderness environment, removed from urban spaces, the second is a green space in a built-up area, like a park, and the last is an indoor, built green space. While all three can help to reduce tension, wild places are the most beneficial, so it's a good idea to make the extra effort occasionally to take a camping trip or a long hike.

Benefits of Being in Nature More Often

So, if being in nature fundamentally changes our brains, what benefits will you reap?

First and foremost, it heals, soothes, and restores you. It's physically healing for us to even see nature, and studies have shown that just viewing scenes of nature can help to reduce negative emotions such as anxiety, fear, and anger (Berman et al., 2008). Exposure to natural space also soothes our bodies and minds, helping us to deal with pain. This is because it both distracts us and reduces stress, making us feel positive. Lastly, it restores and reinvigorates us, boosting the ability of our consciousness to operate and making our bodies feel rejuvenated.

Studies have also shown that being in nature can help you to both reduce and manage mood disorders such as anxiety and depression (Yar & Thorpe, 2020). It doesn't have to be a major hiking mission into the unknown to produce this benefit; something as simple as a daily walk can achieve it. Linked to this, nature can greatly reduce feelings of pressure because our bodies release less cortisol when we are in nature, and we feel like we finally have a chance to breathe. Our cognitive functioning is boosted, and regular forays into the great outdoors have also been shown to increase the quality of your sleep.

Ways to Increase Your Exposure to Nature

If you don't currently spend any time in nature, it can be daunting to try and find a way to fit it into your current lifestyle. However, it's vital that you do. You don't have to start big and run into the woods tomorrow for a five-day hike. Start small, be consistent, and build your way up. Eventually, you will find that you start to crave these moments outside.

Start simple and aim to take short walks a few times a week. Try and find a park to walk to near your house or some other small green space. This is a convenient and accessible way to get a little but important dose of the outside a few times a week. You could also switch up your current schedule to incorporate some more outdoor time. If you're close enough to your place of work, you could wake up slightly earlier and walk or bike to work to get some fresh air. You could also choose to do your workouts outside instead of at home or the gym, and many gyms even have equipment that can be used outside. You could plan nature dates with your friends or partner. The next time you plan a social date, make it an outside event. Go to the beach instead of the mall, or go for a picnic in the local park instead of going to a cafe for lunch. Another terrific option is to set aside time to meditate outdoors, giving your mind a double dose of mindfulness and a bit of nature. Just doing this in your garden could have a lot of benefits, but finding a park and taking half an hour to meditate and journal in the fresh air surrounded by green will have a colossal impact on the way you feel.

While it might be harder to find time to spend in the wilder outdoors, there are also ways to make it easier. One way is to find a group or a nature buddy, a friend of yours who also wants to venture outside a bit more, and further afield. It's far more motivating when you have someone to do something with, and you're less likely to give up if someone else is holding you accountable. As an added bonus, you get your socializing in too! Maybe even pick an outdoor activity together that you want to take up from scratch. It can be hiking, climbing, swimming, stand-up paddleboarding, or kayaking—whatever you want! Try a few and see what you like. Building skill is far more motivating when you enjoy it.

Spending more time connecting with the earth is an essential part of decluttering your mind, and while it might be harder to find time to incorporate this strategy, it's not one you should skip.

Strategy Summary: Get Outside

Our bodies thrive when we give them time outdoors—both mentally and physically. Being in nature soothes and heals us, boosts our well-being, and gives our brains a break from everyday stress. It's a crucial part of decluttering your mind and boosting your brain power.

12

Strategy #8: Practice Gratitude

The phrase "stop and smell the roses" is commonplace because it actually holds a lot of wisdom. When we are very busy, we often feel overwhelmed, stressed, and anxious, and the thought of slowing down seems like the worst idea because of the fear of falling even further behind. But taking moments for yourself and slowing down your pace is important because it allows you to stop and take stock of your life and all the things you have to be grateful for.

When we practice gratitude, it's far harder for our minds to be cluttered with negative thoughts. So, let's look deeper into what gratitude is, how it works, and the different ways that you can practice it to make it part of your everyday life.

What Is Gratitude?

Gratitude is simply acknowledging all the good things in your life, both big and small. You can have gratitude for the friends and family that make up your social circle, and you can also have gratitude for how happy you feel when you wake up to a sunny day. For some people, gratitude is a part of who they are, they are naturally grateful people. For others, it's a fleeting emotion, they are grateful for something that has happened.

The goal is to cultivate gratitude, to become someone grateful. This allows you to look past the bigger things that are muddling up your mind and be thankful for the good things in your life. When you do this, over time, the negative clutter in your head will disappear.

The Science Behind Gratitude

Practicing gratitude works not only because it feels good emotionally, but also because it alters our brain on a chemical level. Studies have shown that practicing gratitude over extended periods strengthens the brain's neural circuits for practicing gratitude, meaning that once you develop the habit, your brain will start to do it unconsciously (Burton, 2016). So if you remind yourself every morning that you are grateful for your hot cup of coffee and the warmth it brings you, your mind will take note of that hot coffee every morning, and the feeling of gratitude will come back. This becomes an antidote to negative emotions when your brain starts to automatically seek out positive things for you.

Practicing gratitude has also been shown to lead to increased dopamine and serotonin production, which are the neurochemicals that help us to feel happy. Serotonin has been dubbed "the happy chemical" and dopamine is responsible for allowing us to feel positive emotions such as motivation, pleasure, and reward (Lechner, 2019). When dopamine is increased, we feel a natural high; and when it's produced consistently, we experience positive emotions for longer. Serotonin also helps to regulate our feelings, usually leading to less anxiety and more contentment and happiness. Furthermore, explicitly expressing gratitude increases activity in our medial prefrontal cortex, which is the part of the brain linked to learning and decision-making, so expressing your gratitude to those around you can boost your cognitive skills. It also activates the part of your brain that responds to altruism, and this means that gratitude can also make you more selfless and charitable.

Therefore, practicing gratitude will stimulate and boost the parts of your brain that help you to feel happy, stable, and balanced.

Benefits of Practicing Gratitude

The happiness and reward centers of our brain are stimulated when we practice gratitude, and this can lead to several benefits.

However, it goes far beyond that. An increase in positive thoughts releases us from the terrifying grip of negative emotions. We only have so much room in our thoughts, and when we spend time focusing on positive things, there is far less space for us to focus on negative feelings of insecurity, resentment, or envy. Together with this and increased serotonin release, practicing gratitude is shown to have a significant effect on reducing feelings of depression. This is also because gratitude alters the structure of the area of the brain that is linked to depression (Fox, 2019). The dopamine that gratitude releases also tends to reduce pressure, as cortisol production is also inhibited, and reduces feelings of pain.

As you can see, gratitude leaves a significant impression on our brains, and it's not some fleeting change, but a long-lasting shift. As previously mentioned, when we practice gratitude consistently, the medial prefrontal cortex shows an increased amount of activity, serotonin and dopamine increase, and the altruistic part of our brain is also stimulated. These changes do not fade over time, but rather strengthen. Going forward, you will find yourself routinely happier and more stable, more eager to give and be charitable, and your cognitive skills will stay consistently sharp. Gratitude leaves a permanent impression on our minds. Outside of our emotions, gratitude has been shown to help improve our overall health too.

Ways to Practice Gratitude

It's important to note that you don't need to publicly announce what you are grateful for to reap the benefits of practicing gratitude, it can be something you do just for yourself. It's important to realize, however, that the effects of practicing gratitude take time. This is not a quick fix or something you will feel immediately. As you go along, you will notice more and more benefits, but this will happen only if you're consistent and persistent. Find ways to practice gratitude every day, in small and big ways, and you will find your world vastly improved. Here are some ways you can incorporate gratitude into your everyday life.

Gratitude Journals and Letters

Gratitude journals are one of the most popular ways to practice gratitude. This habit is exactly as it sounds; you keep a journal that you use once or twice a day to note down all the things that you're grateful for. The key is to be specific, take note of moments with people you love and small joys that bring you happiness. That way, you will easily find a few things to be grateful for every day.

Expressing gratitude to specific people can also be very helpful, and you can do this in the form of a letter. You could write one to people who are no longer in your life, or those closest to you. You can send it to them or just save it for yourself.

Gratitude Meditations

Meditation is often closely linked to gratitude, as it involves taking time in your day to pause and reflect. It's natural that feeling grateful will often come up when you take a quiet moment. You can find guided meditations that specifically focus on gratitude, where someone speaks to you through taking note of what you are grateful for.

Counting Things You Are Grateful For

Another small practice you can do every day is to simply take five minutes in any given room and count out all the things you are grateful for in that space. You might be surprised by how many small things you have to celebrate.

For example, if you were in your kitchen, you could be grateful that you have running water, a fridge full of food, maybe your favorite snack, or a photo on the fridge that makes you happy because it has your family in it. Count all of these up, and slowly make your way through your house; take note of how many small things you have in your space to be thankful for.

Gratitude Jar

A gratitude jar can be a fun way to be crafty as well as practice being grateful. To do this, take a small jar, one that you can spend time decorating in any way that makes you happy, and put it somewhere you see every day, like your bedside table. Each day, take a slip of paper and write down something you are grateful for, then drop it into the jar. If you later have a time when you're feeling overwhelmed or down, open up the jar, and you can read all the things you have to be thankful for.

Strategy Summary: Be Grateful for All That You Have

Gratitude is an excellent practice for decluttering your mind because increasing focus on what you have to be thankful for leaves less space for negative emotions and stress. Studies have shown the extraordinary impact gratitude can have on the way we think, and the benefits are undeniable. It's something that can easily be practiced every day and should be, for a happier and healthier mind and body.

13

Strategy #9: How to Make Better Decisions

One of the greatest problems with mental clutter is how it affects your ability to make decisions, both on a small and a large scale. Whether it's deciding what to have for breakfast, or what you want to do with your life, it can sometimes seem like an insurmountable task to choose something. You may also find that even when you do make decisions, it always seems like the wrong one. This is because mental clutter fogs our brain and slows down our ability to sort through decisions and what needs to be done. Constantly putting off decisions also causes further mental chaos, as the waiting choices remain in the back of your mind until you resolve them.

Learning how to be proactive about the decisions you make is a key step in clearing your mind and moving forward because it prevents options from lingering in your mind and taking up space. Reducing your need to make smaller decisions will also clear mental disorder and help you to be more proactive with bigger decisions.

Benefits of Being More Decisive

Being indecisive often stems from insecurity and a lack of confidence. If we believe ourselves to be competent, we generally have an easier time trusting the decisions we make. If you don't already have that sense of confidence, though, you're going to need to fake it until you make it, as they say. One of the benefits of forcing yourself to become more decisive is the self-respect and confidence that you build as a result. Just the act of choosing a path makes us subconsciously feel more sure of ourselves, and feeling like we know what we want builds self-respect. Furthermore, the more you force yourself to be courageous and take charge, the more you will genuinely feel courageous.

When you compel yourself to be proactive in how you make decisions, it also helps you to succeed and embrace failures. Success is a personal thing, and everyone defines it differently, but you can only find success if you learn to make your own decisions. You will never be able to realize your full potential if you cannot be confident in your decisions and what you want. Similarly, you can only fully embrace failure when you become decisive. As a lesson to learn, failure is a key part of success, but if you don't decide to learn from it, it will serve as nothing more than a disappointment.

Lastly, an indecisive life is full of regret. We will always have regrets in life, but if we are timid and cannot make decisions for ourselves, we will inevitably have more regrets than successes.

Ways to Become More Decisive

At this point you may be thinking that being decisive is easier said than done. No matter the benefits, you might still be paralyzed at the thought of making any kind of decision. So how do you push past that?

There are several small ways to press yourself into being more decisive. First, you need to ignore the voice in your head that is desperately trying to see what the 'right' decision is, because there often isn't one. This need to make a perfect choice is often what incapacitates us when we have to make a choice. However, the goal is not to find the so-called right one, as most decisions will lead you to new places and open up new opportunities, regardless of whether you consider your chosen option to be more right or more wrong. The only way to reach those new places and opportunities, though, is to commit to a choice.

Before making a decision, evaluate the long-term impact of each choice. How will this option impact you in a week, a month, or a year? Sometimes you don't know, but other times, it's such a small choice it has no further impact than the next hour. This helps you to focus on the bigger decisions and stop worrying about the small ones. When it comes to bigger decisions, it can also help to think about the outcomes relative to one another to see which one has the potential to bring you more happiness. You can never be certain, but it's always likely that one that has the potential for more happiness than the other does. If you feel you cannot accurately do this yet, is there any way for you to gather more information about each decision that would help to increase your confidence in one option or the other? While it may not be directly linked to your happiness, how would it impact your life in other ways? Financially, socially? These are all things you can consider. It's also worth considering if an option needs to be chosen, or whether you could do both, either together or one after the other.

With all that said, while logic is often important in making decisions, sometimes you just have to figure out what your values are and trust your gut. Define what you want in life, what happiness looks like to you, and above all else, what you value. Knowing this will help you to make decisions because you will choose the path that is in line with those values. Furthermore, while there may always be decisions that would be made easier if you had access to information to help you find a path, sometimes you just have to trust your instincts. If you feel your intuition kick in, follow it. Practicing using your natural internal judgement can help you to make confident decisions going forward. While it may be hard to find your inner voice at first, over time it will become clearer to you, and then being decisive will become second nature.

Lastly, and perhaps most importantly, you need to learn to let go of regret. If you spend your time lamenting over the bad choices you have made, it makes it far harder to trust yourself to make choices in the future. While some regret is natural, you don't need to stew in it. Try and learn from it, and then keep moving forward.

Reduce Your Daily Need to Make Decisions

While being proactive in your decision-making is an important part of taming mental chaos, finding ways to reduce the number of decisions you make is also important for clearing your mind's clutter. It's important to be proactive when you're making big decisions, but to help with this you need to reduce the number of small decisions you are forced to make every day.

We can reach a place where we suffer what is known as "decision fatigue" where we have made so many choices that our minds cannot do any more, we have used up all of our will. If you wake up with no plan, and you are therefore deciding everything in your day from what workout to do, to which fruit to top your oatmeal with, your brain runs out of fuel to make decisions when it comes to the bigger issues. Therefore, by making the smaller decisions in life routine, you can reduce fatigue.

The key is to put unimportant things on autopilot. So instead of deciding each morning whether you're going to work out, just do it; don't make it optional. If you have a set workout plan each week, you don't have to decide what workout you are going to do. Instead of choosing what you're going to wear each morning, have a few set outfits that you just repeat. Instead of trying to decide what to cook and eat each day, plan all your meals for the week on Sunday.

By taking away all of these small decisions, you have more willpower to be decisive for the important things. Furthermore, these less significant decisions just clutter your mind until you resolve them, so taking them away helps to clear your head, making hard decisions easier to make.

Strategy Summary: Become Decisive

Living indecisively and making continual, small decisions fills your mind with useless and unavoidable clutter. To work through this, you need to learn to be more proactive and confident in your decisions. Reducing the number of small decisions you make in a day both clears clutter and makes it easier for you to make proactive decisions.

14

Strategy #10: Create Healthy Habits and Routines

The key to any lifestyle change is making your new way of a life a habit and making it part of your normal daily routine. When you have a healthy routine, you don't have to do anything, it just becomes second nature. Furthermore, having a routine boosts your mental health and keeps your mind clear, bringing a certainty and structure to your life that enables you to thrive.

The Mental Health Benefits of Creating a Daily Routine

Having a simple everyday or weekly routine is highly beneficial for good mental health. It can be overwhelming when we have so many things to get done in a day, and they clutter our minds because we have to make so many decisions about when to do what. Routines can help us to contain this stress by having a set order that we tackle things every day. These habits alleviate anxiety, as doing things every day helps them to become easier over time. It allows you to be productive without having to think about it.

Routines are also important for us to develop healthy habits. As we discussed in Chapter 3, a healthy lifestyle is essential for good mental health and clearing clutter. It's far easier to maintain habits of exercising, healthy eating, and a regular sleeping pattern if we make it part of our routine. Maybe you do this by waking up early to work out and making sure you can go to bed at a good time every night. Maybe you always make extra at dinner so you can have a healthy lunch the following day. Creating little routines like this is essential for developing a healthy lifestyle. In fact, a regular routine is essential for improving your sleep, as you should be going to sleep and waking up at the same time every day. Good evening and morning practices will help with this, as you are less likely to lie around in bed if you have a set routine you know you need to do when you wake up. This also helps you to start your day off right because being productive in the first few hours of the morning tends to boost your mood because you have accomplished something early.

Routines also combat burnout by allowing you to get everything done while still having time for yourself and your personal priorities. They give your life structure that prevents you from feeling overwhelmed and reduce the daily pressure that comes from having unorganized days. Routines foster good mental health because they are predictable and calming, while change is stressful and not something our minds or bodies handle well. Waking up and knowing exactly what you need to do and how to do it will great reduce your level of stress. Additionally, as we discussed in the previous chapter, having a set routine when you wake up also reduces decision fatigue, meaning you are proactively able to make more important decisions.

Creating routines also ensures that you can do all the things you need to do in a day, while still having time for what makes you happy, like hobbies, relaxation, and spending time with family and friends. Having the opportunity to do this is important for reducing pressure and will help you to sustain routines and healthy habits.

Simple Daily Habits You Can Adopt

In the beginning, it can be hard to develop and maintain new habits, especially when you try to change everything all at once. Your body and mind are averse to change, and making a lot of major modifications in your life at once can actually cause more harm than good. You should therefore pick a few small habits to start off with. Try to make two or three adjustments to your practices each week until you build up to a sustainable routine.

After all, they say a habit is formed in 21 days, and that's just three weeks of being consistent. So, let's look at some sustainable ways you can start small:

Wake Up Early and Go to Bed Early

It doesn't need to be dark, but waking up at a fairly early hour is essential for optimal health. In fact, most natural pattern to match our circadian rhythm is to wake up when the sun rises and go to bed when the sun sets. Therefore, going to bed early and waking up early are both great habits to adopt, and they will also allow you to get enough sleep.

Drink Water When You Wake Up

Hydration is essential for the maintenance of a healthy body, but it can be hard to go from drinking very little water in a day to two liters every day immediately. To start slowly, just commit to drinking a glass of water as soon as you wake up. It wouldn't be a big leap from that to then having another glass of water just before bed, and then you will have easily introduced a very healthy new adjustment to your daily activities.

Spend Time Outside

As we explored in Chapter 11, spending time in nature is one of the best natural remedies for our bodies and our minds, and one that is easily accessible. You don't need to venture out on a great adventure to reap the benefits, rather you can start by spending only 10 minutes outside every day, getting some vitamin D, and breathing in the fresh air.

Cook Healthy Meals and Eat Mindfully

In Chapter 3, we looked at the importance of eating a balanced and nourishing diet. The only way to do this sustainably is to cook for yourself. It doesn't have to be gourmet quality, but doing your own cooking ensures you are getting all the correct nutrients and that you are consuming whole foods, free from preservatives. Commit to cooking one healthy meal for yourself each day, and make a lot so it can become leftovers, too, and solve a meal decision for another day.

It's also important to develop good eating habits. When we eat in front of the TV or while scrolling through our phones, we are not eating mindfully, and it does not nourish or fill us up in the same way. Make a habit of sitting down for every meal and focus just on eating with no distractions. Savor every bite and you will feel the difference.

Make Time to Move Your Body

Again, we refer back to Chapter 3 and the long list of benefits that exercise has for both your mental and physical health. When it comes to building an exercise routine, if you're not already accustomed to regular exercise, then it's definitely better to start off slowly and try to just move your body once a day. Maybe it's a workout, or maybe you go for a slow walk or just stretch for 10 minutes. What's important is that you make time for something every day in order to build the consistent habit that will make it part of your normal routine.

Put Away Your Phone and Start Reading

As we explored when looking at digital detoxing, any time away from our devices is good for our mental health. It's important to make time for it in your everyday routine, and it is an easy habit to introduce. Start by putting away your phone for one hour before you go to sleep. Then over time, extend it until your whole evening is device-free.

Another beneficial habit to initiate is reading—it expands your mind, decreases stress, and makes you feel productive. To start off, commit to reading only 10 pages a day, and if you find it difficult to do that, then start with only five; you can do it in the hour before you sleep when your phone is put away! Start with a book that excites you and is easy to get into. Once it has become a habit, you can pick books that challenge you more.

Finding a Daily Routine That Suits You and Optimizes Your Mind

All routines are beneficial, but you will find that you enjoy and benefit from some routines more than others. While you can find specific guidelines and examples online, the best routine for you will be one that you have personalized and created for yourself.

To create your routine, first you need to make a list. This will just be a kind of brain dump, so it doesn't have to be perfect. Just write down everything you need to do as well as everything you want to get done in a day.

Then, structure your day around when you are most productive. Some people tend to race through tasks in the morning and crash in the afternoon, while others are slow in the morning and find they are more productive later in the day. So, put the laborious but mindless tasks in the part of the day when you are least productive, like working out or doing household chores, and save your work for when your brain is sharp. This will help you make the most of your time.

As you plan your routine, be specific. If you wish, you can record everything down to the last fine detail, such as setting aside 15 minutes to brush your teeth and wash your face. When you start, planning down to the minute can help you to get the hang of it. However, it's also important to be flexible; and incidents like doctor's appointments and social activities need to be able to fit into your routine when they crop up.

Give yourself time to adjust to your new pattern of activity, and if something is not working, change it! Play around with it and see what works best for you; but make sure your routine is something that is reducing stress and helping you to thrive instead of adding extra anxiety.

Three Questions to Ask Yourself Every Day

To end every day, ask yourself the following questions to gauge where you are and clear your mind of any clutter that has accumulated. This is a good way to end your routine and unload any anxieties from your head.

Am I Doing What I Love?

This one is simple enough—is what you are doing day to day making you happy and fulfilled? If today was your last day, would you be happy with what you did? You will only reach your best self by making sure you can answer 'yes' to this question every day.

What's the Worst That Could Happen?

This question is designed to stop your anxiety from running wild. It's natural to be worried about the future, about where you're going, but usually that worry has little benefit and serves only to create pressure. So, make a point every day to stop and ask yourself, what is the worst that could happen, really? When you do pin down exactly what the worst-case scenario might be, it's often not actually all that bad, so this can be a good way to quell and clear anxieties that linger in the back of your consciousness.

What Good Have I Done Today?

This question allows you to reflect, take a moment, and wonder what you are doing for the world. Helping others and doing good will give you a sense of purpose and contentment. Simply recognizing the difference you have made in your own life or someone else's can create a sense of gratitude and the pause that your brain needs to sweep away the clutter.

Strategy Summary: Routines and Habits Are Important

Our minds and body struggle when they are subject to constant change, so routines are important not only because they help us to create healthy habits, but also because they reduce stress and anxiety. They are an important part of clearing clutter from your head by making your everyday life more simple and straightforward.

Conclusion

Mental clutter holds us back in so many ways. It slows down our minds, makes us foggy, anxious, and stressed. Like an overloaded physical space, we often don't realize how much a crowded mind is holding us back until we stop and take the time to clear it out again. Moving through life feeling heavy, tired, and constantly pressurized is not natural and decreases the quality of our lives significantly.

If you follow through with all the strategies outlined in this book, you will be able to make changes so that you won't have to live like that any longer.

While the strategies discussed happen externally, decluttering your mind is a very internal process. It's about sitting in your mind and consciously recognizing what is lingering there that you need to keep and what is harming you. It's a lifestyle change that does not need much to be successful, it doesn't require a lot of time or a new gym membership. By simply taking a few moments out of your everyday life to work through these strategies, you will notice an immense difference. You will have an increased level of energy and vitality for life because the things that once weighed you down mentally will be gone. You will find yourself feeling lighter, less worn down with persistent pressure, anxiety, or feelings of depression. Concentration and focus will come quicker to you.

Because you have read through all the advice in this book, you already have the power to make this change. Unconsciously, you will have already started on the journey. By reading through the actions that you need to address, you will have picked up on negative thought patterns that you practice and already started to fight against them. You will already have found yourself practicing gratitude in smaller ways, noticing little things in your day that make you happy. As you put down this book, it's time to actively start the process, so pick one or two strategies and start with them immediately. Maybe when you wake up tomorrow, you can start the first day of your gratitude journal or start a plan to declutter the various rooms in your house. If you feel overwhelmed, just commit to 20 minutes every day starting tomorrow. There is no rush to clear your mind, you can take it at any pace. The key is to do it well, rather than to race through it.

A happier, easier, and more fulfilling life is easily within your reach. All you have to do is look inward and get rid of the things that you are carrying around that will not lead you to that life. But you have already taken the first step, now all you have to do is keep your momentum going.

***

Thank you for taking the time to read Detox Our Brain. I hope that you have enjoyed reading it as much as I have enjoyed writing it. I would be very grateful if you could leave me a review on Amazon or at **www.magletpublishing.com** to help others realize the benefits of having a brain detox every now and again. Just scan the QR code below.

If you'd like to download a free Wheel of Life template to help you assess areas in your life that might need some work, head over to: www.magletpublishing.com/wheeloflife

Other books in the Things We Need To Do series:

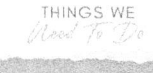
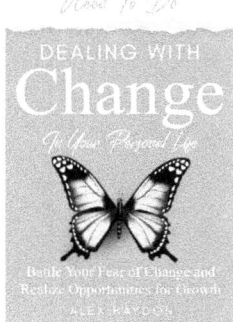
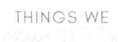
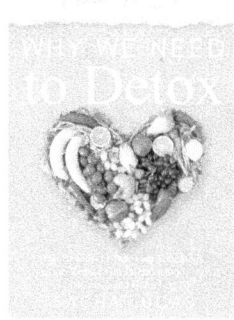
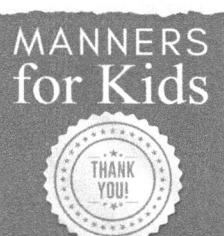

Author Bio

My name is Sacha Lucas, and I am passionate about helping others to achieve the level of happiness that I have found through decluttering.

I was struggling through life in my early 30s, stressed, overwhelmed, and just completely lost. Then I stopped for a moment, focused on my health and found my way back. I am passionate about guiding people through the same process by helping them take back their minds and their bodies through decluttering.

Bibliography

Berman, M. G., Jonides, J., & Kaplan, S. (2008). The cognitive benefits of interacting with nature. Psychological Science, 19(12), 1207–1212. https://doi.org/10.1111/j.1467-9280.2008.02225.x

Burton, L. R. (2016, October). The neuroscience of gratitude. Wharton Health Care Management Alumni Association. https://www.whartonhealthcare.org/the_neuroscience_of_gratitude

Centers for Disease Control and Prevention. (2020). How much physical activity do adults need? Centers for Disease Control and Prevention. https://www.cdc.gov/physicalactivity/basics/adults/index.htm

Cherry, K. (2019). The benefits of doing a digital detox. Verywell Mind. https://www.verywellmind.com/why-and-how-to-do-a-digital-detox-4771321

Drew, D. R. (2020, July 24). Glymphatic system and trying to get enough sleep. Specialized Therapy. https://www.specializedtherapy.com/the-glymphatic-system-and-sleep/

Emmons, R., (2010, November 16). Why Gratitude Is Good. Great Good Magazine. https://greatergood.berkeley.edu/article/item/why_gratitude_is_good

Fox, G. (2019, June 10). What science reveals about gratitude's impact on the brain. Mindful. https://www.mindful.org/what-the-brain-reveals-about-gratitude/

Goyal, M., Singh, S., Sibinga, E. M. S., Gould, N. F., Rowland-Seymour, A., Sharma, R., Berger, Z., Sleicher, D., Maron, D. D., Shihab, H. M., Ranasinghe, P. D., Linn, S., Saha, S., Bass, E. B., & Haythornthwaite, J. A. (2014). Meditation programs for psychological stress and well-being. JAMA Internal Medicine, 174(3), 357. https://doi.org/10.1001/jamainternmed.2013.13018

Jessen, N. A., Munk, A. S. F., Lundgaard, I., & Nedergaard, M. (2015). The glymphatic system: A beginner's guide. Neurochemical Research, 40(12), 2583–2599. https://doi.org/10.1007/s11064-015-1581-6

Killgore, W. D. S. (2010). Effects of sleep deprivation on cognition. Progress in Brain Research. https://pubmed.ncbi.nlm.nih.gov/21075236/

Lechner, T. (2019, November 26). The neuroscience behind gratitude: How does cultivating appreciation affect your brain? The Chopra Center. https://chopra.com/articles/the-neuroscience-behind-gratitude-how-does-cultivating-appreciation-affect-your-brain

Legg, T. J. (2018, June 1). Box breathing: How to do it, benefits, and tips. Www.medicalnewstoday.com. https://www.medicalnewstoday.com/articles/321805#benefits

Liao, W.-C., Landis, C. A., Lentz, M. J., & Chiu, M.-J. (2005). Effect of foot bathing on distal-proximal skin temperature gradient in elders. International Journal of

Nursing Studies, 42(7), 717–722. https://doi.org/10.1016/j.ijnurstu.2004.11.011

Mann, D. (2009, December 30). Sleep and weight gain. WebMD. https://www.web-md.com/sleep-disorders/features/lack-of-sleep-weight-gain

Marengo, K. (2020, January 2). 12 best brain foods: Memory, concentration, and brain health. Www.medicalnewstoday.com. https://www.medicalnewstoday.-com/articles/324044

Mawer, R. (2020, February 28). 17 proven tips to sleep better at night. Healthline. https://www.healthline.com/nutrition/17-tips-to-sleep-better#5.-Try-to-sleep-and-wake-at-consistent-times

McKay, J. (2020, October 27). Single-tasking: A neuroscientist's guide to doing one thing at a time. RescueTime Blog. https://blog.rescuetime.com/single-tasking/

Mergenthaler, P., Lindauer, U., Dienel, G. A., & Meisel, A. (2013). Sugar for the brain: the role of glucose in physiological and pathological brain function. Trends in Neurosciences, 36(10), 587–597. https://doi.org/10.1016/j.tins.2013.07.001

Meyer, D. (2020, April 18). What is mental clutter? (and how to clear it). Simple Not Stressful. https://simplenotstressful.com/blog/mental-clutter

Newman, T. (2019, June 21). The glymphatic system: What is it and what does it do? Www.medicalnewstoday.com. https://www.medicalnewstoday.com/arti-cles/325493#The-importance-of-sleep

Oshin, M. (2018, September 10). 9 ways multitasking is killing your brain and productivity, according to neuroscientists. Ladders | Business News & Career Advice. https://www.theladders.com/career-advice/9-ways-multitasking-is-killing-your-brain-and-productivity-according-to-neuroscientists

Reeves, Benjamin C., Karimy, Jason K., Kundishora, Adam J., Mestre, H., Cerci, H Mert, Matouk, Charles, Alper, Seth L., Lundgaard, Iben, Nedergaard, Maiken, & Kahle, Kristopher T. (2020, March). Glymphatic System Impairment in Alzheimer's Disease and Idiopathic Normal Pressure Hydrocephalus, Trends in Molecular Medicine, 26(3), 285-295.

Roster, C., Ferrari, J., & Jurkat, M. (2016, March). The dark side of home: Assessing possession "clutter" on subjective well-being. ResearchGate. https://www.re-searchgate.net/publication/298428874_The_dark_side_of_home_Assess-ing_possession_

Twohig-Bennett, C., & Jones, A. (2018). The health benefits of the great outdoors: A systematic review and meta-analysis of greenspace exposure and health outcomes. Environmental Research, 166(3), 628–637. https://doi.org/10.1016/j.envres.2018.06.030

van de Rest, O., Berendsen, A. A., Haveman-Nies, A., & de Groot, L. C. (2015). Dietary patterns, cognitive decline, and dementia: A systematic review. Advances in Nutrition, 6(2), 154–168. https://doi.org/10.3945/an.114.007617

Vartanian, L. R., Kernan, K., & Wansink, B. (2016). Clutter, chaos, and overconsumption: the role of mind-set in stressful and chaotic food environments. SSRN Electronic Journal, 49(2). https://doi.org/10.2139/ssrn.2711870

Walton, A. G. (2016, December 9). 7 ways sleep affects the brain (and what happens if it doesn't get enough). Forbes. https://www.forbes.com/sites/alicegwalton/2016/12/09/7-ways-sleep-affects-the-brain-and-what-happens-if-it-doesnt-get-enough/?sh=6d22ffbd753c

Walton, A. G. (2019, February 9). 7 ways meditation can actually change the brain. Forbes. https://www.forbes.com/sites/alicegwalton/2015/02/09/7-ways-meditation-can-actually-change-the-brain/?sh=4a3e4cb14658

Yar, S., & Thorpe, J. (2020, May 29). 5 ways being in nature changes your brain, according to science. Bustle. https://www.bustle.com/p/5-ways-being-in-nature-changes-your-brain-according-to-science-15827469